Internet of Medical Things

The book presents a comprehensive overview of emerging IoT technologies, IoT devices, and sensors and their role in the healthcare industry. It offers recent developments in the creation, application, and security of IoMT data, as well as various IoMT devices used in applications including telemedicine, monitoring patients, and artificial intelligence-based medical data analysis. It includes discussions on the use of medical data analysis to make various predictions and diagnoses that lead to the right treatment. The security of medical data from Internet of Things (IoT) devices, where there is a risk of data leakage during transmission from the device to the server, is also discussed. The book:

- Offers Software Application Framework for Sustainable Healthcare.
- Includes feature case studies and real-world examples of IoT devices and technologies in use in healthcare settings.
- Provides insight into the security risks associated with connected medical devices and the measures that can be taken to mitigate these risks.
- Discusses various integration strategies and technologies, including data. interoperability standards, application programming interfaces (APIs), and other tools.
- Contains discussions on emerging IoT technologies, such as blockchain and edge computing, as well as their potential applications in healthcare.

This book is for researchers, professionals, and students interested in the latest advancements on Internet of Medical Things.

Internet of Medical Things

Case Studies and Applications in Healthcare

Edited by
Balakrishnan C, Jayapriya J, Vinay M,
Sanjeev Kumar Singh, and
Nadarajah Manivannan

CRC Press
Taylor & Francis Group
Boca Raton London New York

CRC Press is an imprint of the
Taylor & Francis Group, an **informa** business
A CHAPMAN & HALL BOOK

Designed cover image: ShutterStock

First edition published 2026
by CRC Press
2385 NW Executive Center Drive, Suite 320, Boca Raton FL 33431

and by CRC Press
4 Park Square, Milton Park, Abingdon, Oxon, OX14 4RN

CRC Press is an imprint of Taylor & Francis Group, LLC

Library of Congress Cataloging-in-Publication Data
Names: C, Balakrishnan editor | J, Jayapriya editor | Vinay, M. editor |
Singh, Sanjeev Kumar (Professor of bioinformatics) editor | Manivannan,
Nadarajah editor
Title: Internet of medical things : case studies and applications in
healthcare / edited by Balakrishnan C, Jayapriya J, Vinay M, Sanjeev
Kumar Singh, Nadarajah Manivannan.
Description: First edition. | Boca Raton: C&H/CRC Press, 2026. |
Includes bibliographical references and index. | Summary: "The book presents a
comprehensive overview of emerging IoT technologies, IoT devices and sensors and their
role in the healthcare industry. It offers recent developments in the creation, application, and
impact of new IoMT data security, IoMT devices used in a variety of applications, including
telemedicine, monitoring patients, and intelligence-based medical data analysis.
It includes discussions on the use of medical data analysis to make various predictions and
diagnoses that lead to the right treatment. The security of medical data from Internet of Things (IoT) devices,
where there is a risk of data leakage during transmission from the device to the server,
is also discussed. Offers Software Application Framework for Sustainable Healthcare
Includes feature case studies and real-world examples of IoT devices and technologies in use in healthcare
settings Provide insight into the security risks associated with connected medical devices and the
measures that can be taken to mitigate these risks. Discusses various integration strategies and technologies,
including data interoperability standards, application programming interfaces (APIs), and other
tools Contains discussions on emerging IoT technologies, such as blockchain and edge computing,
as well as their potential applications in healthcare This book is for researchers, professionals
and students interested in the latest advancements on Internal of Medical Things"-- Provided by publisher.
Identifiers: LCCN 2025028380 (print) | LCCN 2025028381 (ebook) | ISBN 9781032748931 hbk |
ISBN 9781032759555 pbk | ISBN 9781003476344 ebk
Subjects: LCSH: Internet of things--Medical applications | Internet of
things--Security measures | Wearable technology--Security measures |
Medical informatics--Security measures
Classification: LCC R859.7.I59 I58 2026 (print) | LCC R859.7.I59 (ebook)
LC record available at https://lccn.loc.gov/2025028380
LC ebook record available at https://lccn.loc.gov/2025028381

ISBN: 978-1-032-74893-1 (hbk)
ISBN: 978-1-032-75955-5 (pbk)
ISBN: 978-1-003-47634-4 (ebk)

DOI: 10.1201/ 9781003476344

Typeset in Times
by Deanta Global Publishing Services, Chennai, India

Contents

Foreword

I offer this foreword to the timely and necessary contribution to the growing field of health technology: a comprehensive exploration of the Internet of Medical Things (IoMT). When we stand in the abyss of Healthcare 4.0, the concepts and advances described in these pages are not just theoretical discussions but the futuristic blueprint of patients' care, remote medical assistance, and personal health empowerment. Sophisticated medical devices and cloud platforms from wearable sensors, how to activate the flow of seamless data, how the diagnoses are done, treatment is performed, and the well-being of the patients is constantly monitored. Only economic indicators, the best market is already valuable as a vision and is planned for exponential growth. This revolution has an undeniable momentum. However, the completely composite and optimized IoMT ecosystem pathway is filled with complex challenges, the most important of which is the main concern of data safety.

The inherent sensitivity of medical information calls for firm attention to the defensive frameworks against cyber threats. This book resolves with the correct ranking, exploring advanced cryptographic solutions and enhanced data integrity and blockchain applications for confidentiality. Furthermore, the thoughtful exploration of IoMT on mental health and mental well-being is especially related to our increasingly complex world. The book emphasizes the human-centered ability of technology by checking that IoMT systems can equip natural language processing (NLP) for personalized interventions for telecommunications, depression, and other conditions. It thinks of moral dimensions, privacy concerns, and the ability of social inequalities, we must carefully navigate when we combine IoM into a variety of communities.

Finally, the book is higher than the technical book. This is a healthy, more connected future vision. The authors have created a precious resource for researchers, doctors, policymakers, and anyone who wants to understand the in-depth effects of IoMT. It is not only a snapshot of the current progress but also gives an understanding of a foundation that conveys and inspires future innovations. I appreciate the authors for their perceptive contributions and endorse this book with a full heart as a vital guide for the opening of medical technology.

Dr Fr Jossy P George
Director, Bannerghatta Road Campus
CHRIST (Deemed to be University)
Bengaluru, Karnataka, India

Preface

Healthcare landscape is currently undergoing an unprecedented and most profound transformation, which is often the case with the advent of the Internet of Medical Things (IoMT), which is the revolutionary convergence of inter-sophisticated sensors, sophisticated sensors, and intelligent software, how we approach the care of the patients, and the overall healthcare. The connected healthcare market, valued at $254.20 billion, encompasses a wide range of technologies from sophisticated wearable sensors to complex medical testing equipment. These devices function as intelligent nodes in an expansive network, gathering, transmitting, and aggregating vital medical data to centralized servers. This interconnected system enhances patient care outcomes while providing cost-effective medical solutions. The market is projected to expand at a robust compound annual growth rate (CAGR) of 24.6%. This comprehensive book provides a thorough examination of the Internet of Medical Things (IoMT) and the critical challenges it must overcome to enhance patient health monitoring while managing associated risks. The book begins with an extensive literature review that identifies key research areas, with particular attention to security concerns. The book explores IoMT's compound architectural framework, probing the foundational infrastructure that allows seamless communication and integration across diverse healthcare technologies. This includes wearable devices, embedded sensors, medical imaging equipment, cloud-based platforms, and Electronic Health Records (EHR) systems, all intended to provision real-time data processing while upholding scalability, security, and interoperability.

The book covers advanced sensing technologies that permit the incessant assortment of dynamic health data, as well as the communication protocols that confirm efficient and secure data transmission all over the network. Additionally, it examines the transformative role of Artificial Intelligence (AI) and Machine Learning (ML) in analyzing extensive healthcare datasets to support disease diagnosis, develop personalized treatment strategies, and enable predictive maintenance of medical equipment. Through this multifaceted approach, the book offers valuable insights into optimizing IoMT systems for improved healthcare delivery. The book specifies uses of IoMT and illustrates its adaptability in a variety of medical fields. Using a cutting-edge smart system to gather extensive data and produce in-depth reports on patterns and quality, a noteworthy case study is given. It has significant ability to identify, leading to advanced, non-invasive diagnostic devices. Essentially, the Internet of Medical Things is not just a technological advancement, but also a true converter of health and patient care. This book aims to provide a comprehensive overview of IoMT architecture, including its foundation and modification.

The editors express sincere gratitude to the administration and colleagues of CHRIST University, Alagappa University, and Brunel University, UK, for invaluable encouragement and support during the compilation of this book and the collection of contributed chapters from various esteemed authors. Additionally, the editors deeply appreciate the continuous moral support provided by their family members throughout this endeavor. Special thanks are also extended to CRC Press officials, whose consistent support, guidance, and assistance were instrumental since the initial acceptance of the proposal through to the final publication stage. Furthermore, heartfelt thanks are extended to Dr. Mahalakshmi J., Assistant Professor; Shubhi Jain, BCA student; and Prathish R.K. and Nileem Kaveramma, M.Sc. (Data Science) students, from the Department of Computer Science, CHRIST University—Bangalore Yeshwanthpur Campus, for their dedicated efforts and assistance in collecting and organizing the chapters.

Balakrishnan C.
Jayapriya J.
Vinay M.
Sanjeev Kumar Singh
Nadarajah Manivannan

Editor Biography

Balakrishnan C. is Associate Professor of Computer Science at CHRIST University (Deemed to be University), Bengaluru, India. Formerly, he was teaching in Alagappa University, Karaikudi, and St. Joseph's College, Tiruchirappalli, Tamil Nadu, India. He has 20 years of teaching experience. He obtained his Ph.D. in Computer Science from Bharathidasan University, Tiruchirappalli, India. He has authored 5 books and published more than 50 research articles in international conferences and indexed journals. He has published five Indian patents and contributed to three funded research projects. Presently, he is serving as the coordinator of the prestigious ICSSR Funded Research Programme. His areas of interest are healthcare IoT, vision language models, data analytics, and machine learning.

Jayapriya J. is Assistant Professor in the Department of Computer Science, CHRIST University (Deemed to be University), Bangalore, Karnataka, India. She has 12 years of teaching experience, including working abroad and 5 years of research experience. She completed her Ph.D. at the National Institute of Technology, Tiruchirappalli, India, in 2017. She has published 35+ papers in reputed journals and presented at numerous international conferences. She has also been a reviewer for reputed journals and acted as a resource person for many workshops and seminars. She specializes in computational intelligence, bioinformatics, cybersecurity, and data science. She completed a project funded by the Australian Consulate and is currently working on an ICSSR project. She is a member of IEEE, CS, and WIE.

Vinay M. is an academic and a researcher with a distinguished career spanning nearly two decades. Currently serving as the Head of the Department at CHRIST (Deemed to be University), his expertise lies in the fields of artificial intelligence (AI) and Information and Communication Technology (ICT). He is a Google Certified Trainer. His research interests encompass cutting-edge domains such as generative AI, virtual reality (VR), augmented reality (AR), and cybersecurity. He has published 25 research papers indexed in Scopus and has participated in 30+ conferences. His contributions to the field have been recognized with 3 Best Paper Awards. His expertise extends beyond research, and he served as a resource person for over 150 academic programs, sharing knowledge and insights with various audiences. He is a member of the Institute of Electrical and Electronics Engineers (IEEE) and is involved in numerous projects.

Sanjeev Kumar Singh is Professor in the Department of Bioinformatics, Alagappa University, Tamil Nadu, India. He received his Ph.D. in Applied Chemistry from CJSM University, Kanpur, in 2004. He holds several administrative positions in different capacities within the university. He has vast experience of 20 years in research/teaching and has published more than 250 international and national research articles/reviews/book chapters in peer-reviewed journals. His outstanding research in

HIV integrates and protease has been recognized by the Indian Council of Medical Research (ICMR) through the honor of ICMR Lala Ram Chand Kandhari Award for the year 2014. He has also received several awards and honors in research career: Fellow of Royal Society of Chemistry from the Royal Society of Chemistry, London, UK, for the outstanding contribution in the field of molecular modeling and computer-aided drug design with quantum chemistry applications, Fellow of Royal Society of Biology from the Royal Society of Biology, London, UK, for the extensive research involved in the field of biological sciences, Member of Board of Governors (2021–2023) for the Biotech Research Society of India (BRSI), India. Dr. Singh's research interests include neutralizing the HIV infection by targeting different proteins crucial for the virus' existence. He is keenly interested in investigating small molecules that exclusively interact with CDKs, HAT, h-GPCR, retinoblastoma, and HPV to potentially aid therapeutics.

Nadarajah Manivannan, is Senior Lecturer of Electronics, Computer Languages, and Embedded Systems at the Brunel School of Design. He is associated with Brunel University London for the past 15 years as Researcher and Teaching Faculty. He received his D.Phil. in Optical Pattern Recognition, Electronic Engineering, from the University of Oxford in 1997. Currently, he is working on multiple projects: plasma engineering, microwave plasma, electron gun plasma, emission control, lab-on-chip, optical pattern recognition, and liveness detection of fingerprint biometrics. He is supervising and supporting Ph.D. and M.Sc. students on their research work in the Brunel School of Design. He has to his credit prestigious memberships like Senior Member IEEE, Member of IOP, Member of Oxford Engineering Society, and many more. He contributed in many research projects, like plasma and microwave technologies in emission control funded under DEECON, FP7 EU and MAGS, InnovateUK, optical pattern recognition to explore 4f optical correlator for challenging optical information processing tasks in collaboration with the photonics group at Imperial College, London, fingerprint biometrics for liveness detection of fingerprint, cancelable fingerprint template generation, multi-model biometric fusion techniques, fingerprint in M-health, and many more.

Contributors

Abishek A.
Embedded Systems
U-Blox
Malmö, Sweden

Vaideghy A.
Department of Computer Science
PSG College of Arts and Science
Coimbatore, India

Madalaimuthu Anthony
Department of Psychology
SRM Institute of Science and Technology
Chennai, India

Sundaravadivazhagan Balasubramanian
Department of Information Technology
University of Technology and Applied Sciences
AL Mussanah, Sultanate of Oman

Sujatha Ravinatayana Bhat
College of Banking and Financial Studies
Muscat, Oman

Balakrishnan C.
Department of Computer Science
CHRIST University
Bengaluru, India

Thiyagarajan C.
Department of Computer Science
PSG College of Arts & Science
Coimbatore, India

Suresh Babu C.V.
Department of Information Technology
Hindustan Institute of Technology and Science
Chennai, India

Sonal Devesh
School of Business and Management
CHRIST University
Bengaluru, India

Seshathiri Dhanasekaran
UiT, The Arctic University of Norway
Tromsø, Norway

Abraham Francis
James Cook University
Queensland, Australia

Suruthi G.
Department of Information Technology
Hindustan Institute of Technology and Science
Chennai, India

Rakesh Gnanasekaran
Department of Computer Science
Thiagarajar College
Madurai, India

Devika Govindhan
Department of Computer Science
Mannar Thirumalai Naicker College
Madurai, India

Alberto Ivars-Palomares
Instituto de Investigación para la Gestión Integrada de Zonas Costeras
Universitat Politècnica de València
Valencia, Spain

Mahalakshmi J.
Department of Computer Science
CHRIST University
Bengaluru, India

Jehoson Jiresh J.
Department of English and Cultural Studies
CHRIST University
Bengaluru, India

Jeyakanthan Jeyaraman
Structural Biology and Biocomputing Lab
Department of Bioinformatics
Alagappa University
Karaikudi, India

Ruchi Joshi
Department of Psychology
Manipal University
Jaipur, India

Abarna SriPreethi K.
Independent Researcher
Bengaluru, India

Abilash K.
School of Psychological Sciences
CHRIST University
Bengaluru, India

Mani Abdul Karim
Department of Psychology
XIM University
Bhubaneswar, India

Jaime Lloret
Instituto de Investigación para la Gestión Integrada de Zonas Costeras
Universitat Politècnica de València
Valencia, Spain

Gnanasankaran Natarajan
Department of Computer Science
Thiagarajar College
Madurai, India

Ayisha Nejili
Small Steps Big Dreams
Dubai, UAE

Sindhuja Manisha Kamini P.
Department of Psychology
Alliance University
Bengaluru, India

Sreeja Gangadharan P.
Department of Psychology
CHRIST University
Bengaluru, India

Lorena Parra
Departamento de Producción Agraria
Escuela Técnica Superior de Ingeniería Agronómica
Alimentaria y de Biosistemas
Universidad Politécnica de Madrid
Madrid, Spain

Alphonse P.J.A.
Department of Computer Applications
National Institute of Technology
Tiruchirappalli, India

Sudha R.
Department of Computer Science
PSG College of Arts & Science
Coimbatore, India

Marsha Rodrigues
Department of Psychology
CHRIST University
Bengaluru, India

Soumya R.R.
Department of Psychology
CHRIST University
Bengaluru, India

Baranidharan S.
School of Business and Management
CHRIST University
Bengaluru, India

Kavitha S.
Department of Information Technology
K. Ramakrishnan College of Engineering
Tiruchirappalli, India

Celina Daniel Satyanadan
Department of Psychology
CHRIST University
Bengaluru, India

Sandra Sendra
Instituto de Investigación para la Gestión Integrada de Zonas Costeras
Universitat Politècnica de València
Valencia, Spain

Pradeep Kumar Sriram
Structural Biology and Biocomputing Lab
Department of Bioinformatics
Alagappa University
Karaikudi, India

Maharaja Muthuvairam Subbulakshmi
Structural Biology and Biocomputing Lab
Department of Bioinformatics
Alagappa University
Karaikudi, India

Gomathinayagam Subramanian
Division of Agriculture
University of Guyana
Tain, South America

Alisha Tharwani
Department of Computer Science
CHRIST University
Bengaluru, India

Sandra Viciano-Tudela
Instituto de Investigación para la Gestión Integrada de Zonas Costeras
Universitat Politècnica de València
Valencia, Spain

Gayathry S. Warrier
Department of Computer Science
CHRIST University
Bengaluru, India

Muthu Ramachandran
Forti5 Tech Ltd
London, UK

Introduction

The rapid evolution of technology is ushering in unprecedented change across all sectors, with healthcare at the forefront of this revolution. It marks a paradigm shift towards more effective, customized, and prognostic medical models compared to traditional procedures, often enabled by the Internet of Medical Things (IoMT). The uninterrupted coordination of connected medical devices, sophisticated sensors, and intelligent software is transforming patient care, medical aid, and overall health management.

At its core, IoMT refers to integrating the Internet of Things (IoT) with medical applications. It creates an interconnected system that collects data from medical devices, activates remote monitoring, performs real-time diagnosis, and improves patient care. This growth is paving the way for Healthcare 4.0, which promises more efficient, accessible, and cost-effective medical solutions. From wearable fitness trackers to advanced hospital equipment, IoMT is generating valuable health data, opening new possibilities for preventive care and customized treatment programs. However, this transformation capacity comes with significant challenges, especially regarding data safety and privacy, the central themes discussed throughout this work.

This book reviews essential concepts and key areas required to understand the IoMT landscape:

Architectural Frameworks: Foundational structures that emphasize scalability, real-time processing, and seamless data flow across various units, even for non communicative data sources.

Sensory Systems and Communication Technologies: A detailed overview of sophisticated hardware and communication protocols that facilitate accurate data collection and secure transmission.

Energy Efficiency: Addressing major issues of power management in IoMT devices on a continuous basis.

Artificial Intelligence (AI) and Machine Learning (ML): Exploring how these powerful analytical devices extract functional insights from medical data and how they are driving progress in diagnosis, treatment, and forecast analysis.

Data Safety and Maintenance: Discussion of advanced cryptographic techniques and the role of blockchain technology in protecting sensitive patient information .

Specific Applications: Demonstrating the real-world impact of IoMT implementation and its major role in advancing mental health care from Smart Sleep Monitoring to Smart Sleep Monitoring, as well as its role in the facilities of decentralized clinical experiments.

Sociocultural and Ethical Implications: Examines the broader social impact of the IoMT, including ethical considerations, equity in access, and moral responsibilities related to these technologies.

The book is organized to give logical progress to the concepts of foundation from advanced apps and critical considerations. To begin with, the general issues of IoMT and establishing a research landscape emphasize important challenges such as security. Subsequent chapters systematically build on this foundation, offering separate sections for the integration of architectural units, sensory systems, communication technologies, energy concerns, and AI. It then turns to a detailed exploration of security and data management, and then to a test of specific application cases that display the practical utility of the IOG. The latter parts of the book review the AI, NLP, and IoMT on mental health, which is a climax in the discussion of the broader ethical and moral dimensions that arise from this technical evolution.

To maximize your learning, this book will encourage you to connect the topics systematically. Although each chapter is often designed to be self-contained, sequential reading gives a very elaborate understanding of the correlation of IoMT units and applications. Professionals in health, engineering, computer science, and data analysis can find valuable insights, as well as policymakers with regulatory frameworks. Researchers find a fertile ground for future inquiries, but anyone interested in the future of medicine gets deep appreciation for the converter capacity of the IoMT. This book strives for clarity and accuracy, aimed at entering into complex technical concepts without sacrificing depth.

Our purpose is to provide a balanced and insightful view of IoMT. The range is broad, involving technical grounds and social effects, which ensures a comprehensive understanding of the role of IoT in the evolving health ecosystem. Start this journey with us, because the Internet of Medical Things really redefines how medicine is changing, taking care of health in the 21st century.

1 Introduction to IoMT
A Revolution in Healthcare

Sandra Viciano-Tudela, Alberto Ivars-Palomares, Lorena Parra, Sandra Sendra, and Jaime Lloret

1.1 INTRODUCTION

The evolution of healthcare is undergoing a profound transformation fueled by advancements in smart sensors, artificial intelligence (AI), machine learning (ML), deep learning (DL), the Internet of Medical Things (IoMT), and edge analytics, seamlessly integrated with cloud computing. This interconnected landscape of cutting-edge technologies is capturing widespread attention across industry, government, and healthcare sectors. This innovative paradigm promises to revolutionize healthcare delivery by enabling more precise diagnoses, personalized treatments, and enhanced health management through the seamless integration of devices and medical information systems [1].

The IoMT alleviates healthcare pressure by facilitating early diagnosis [2]. However, preceding IoMT, technologies such as Ambient Assisted Living (AAL) have paved the way for creating safe environments conducive to independent living for assisted individuals [3]. AAL, leveraging ambient intelligence, focuses on preventing, treating, and enhancing health outcomes, particularly in aging populations or those with chronic conditions like diabetes [4]. While AAL addresses specific needs, IoMT emerges as an expansive ecosystem encompassing electronics, sensors, and interconnected devices. IoMT's autonomous data collection, analysis, and medical reporting capabilities offer early and non-intrusive diagnostic possibilities, significantly improving patient outcomes [5].

Central to this transformative healthcare landscape is the concept of patient empowerment. Empowering individuals and communities grants them greater control over decisions impacting their health and well-being. This empowerment entails acquiring diverse skills, accessing information, resources, and influencing factors shaping health outcomes. The World Health Organization (WHO) emphasizes that patient empowerment substantially enhances the quality of healthcare, fostering proactive engagement in one's health journey.

Furthermore, IoMT holds promise beyond conventional medical realms, extending into mental health monitoring. By detecting behavioral patterns through biosignal analysis, IoMT enables remote monitoring of mental health symptoms, offering invaluable insights to healthcare professionals [6]. Addressing mental health is increasingly critical, given its profound societal and economic implications,

DOI: 10.1201/9781003476344-1

particularly among vulnerable populations and those affected by socioeconomic disparities. Understanding the multifaceted determinants of mental health underscores the importance of comprehensive solutions [7].

Aligned with the United Nations' Sustainable Development Goals (SDGs) for 2030, healthcare transformation through IoMT emerges as a strategy in promoting good health and well-being IoMT's potential to enhance healthcare access, diagnostic accuracy, and personalized patient care directly contributes to achieving SDGs related to population health and well-being. As IoMT continues to evolve, it stands poised to redefine healthcare delivery paradigms, driving equitable and sustainable health outcomes for all [8].

1.2 LITERATURE REVIEW

The significant advancement of technology has meant that it is found in all areas. In this way, it integrates with medical devices to enable better treatments, medical solutions, better patient monitoring, and improved personalized healthcare.

After searching for work in the PubMed repository, Figure 1.1 shows the distribution of the six main areas in which research is being carried out, according to Ref. [9]. The study's 129 surveys are included in the Systematic Review, Scheme, Covid, Machine Learning IoMT, and Healthcare System. It is worth highlighting, on the one hand, the importance of IoT in the field of healthcare systems, as 35 surveys

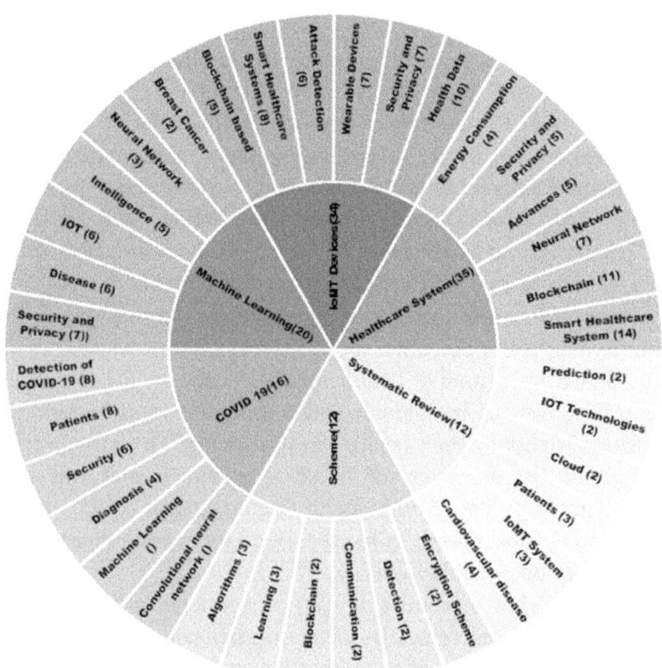

FIGURE 1.1 Summary of current uses of IoMT systems.

have been found. These surveys are distributed into six main topics. On the other hand, in the area of IoMT devices, 34 review articles, which also address six items (blockchains, smart healthcare systems, attack detection, portable devices, security and privacy, and health data), have been found.

Below is an overview of the study topics currently being carried out. In this sense, the concept of the IoMT is established and based on applying technology to the field of medicine. In general, the most discussed topic found in the literature is security in the transmission of medical data, as shown by Hernandez-Jaimes et al. [10], Mahmood et al. [11], Bhushan et al. [12], and Ghubaish et al. [13]. In this case, they focus on collecting work focused on medical data security. They establish a comprehensive overview of the current state of intrusion detection models in Smart Healthcare. They are based on the fact that most attacks are directed at a single type of layer, the network and transport layer of the IoT architecture. There is also talk of collaborative detection based on cloud–fog–edge architectures that allow detection of the first stages of attacks. The different types of algorithms used are asymmetric key algorithms, symmetric key algorithms, and keyless algorithms.

In addition to the security in the treatment and transmission of medical data, the IoMT has been implemented to detect diseases and improve treatments, as shown by Vishnu et al. in 2020 [14]. This study presents an overview of sensor tracking, the treatment of chronic diseases, remote care based on IoT, and smart hospitals.

For the safety and improvement in the treatment of diseases, AI is also applied. Manickam et al., in 2022 [15], reviewed the recent developments and advancements in AI-enabled IoMT devices for efficient disease detection and management. Point-of-care devices are used in cardiac measurement, cancer diagnosis, and diabetes control. In addition, AI is being studied to support robotic surgeries. Ashfaq et al. in 2022 [16] presented a review analyzing the IoMT globally. In it, they present intelligent and remote healthcare monitoring systems. Additionally, they have shown work on wearable and non-wearable sensors, particularly for monitoring patient vital signs.

With this overview, the great relevance of the IoMT is shown, and there is a need to continue developing systems that allow for improving the health system.

1.3 IOMT ARCHITECTURE

The architecture of the IoMT shares similarities with the broader framework of the Internet of Things (IoT), as both define the structural framework governing the interaction and operation of connected devices within their respective systems. In the context of IoMT, this architecture comprises several interconnected layers designed to facilitate seamless communication, data exchange, and intelligent decision-making in healthcare environments.

- Similar to IoT, the first layer of IoMT architecture is the physical/device layer, encompassing sensors, actuators, and other connected smart devices that form the foundational infrastructure. These devices capture vital data from patients, medical equipment, and the surrounding environment.
- The second layer, analogous to IoT's network layer, is the communication layer. It encompasses network devices and protocols such as 5G, Wi-Fi,

and Bluetooth, facilitating the transmission of data between IoMT devices securely and reliably.

- The third layer in IoMT architecture, akin to IoT's data/database layer, manages and stores the vast amounts of data collected by IoMT devices. Designing efficient and secure databases is crucial for storing and accessing the data effectively.
- Moving up the layers, IoMT's fourth layer mirrors IoT's analysis/visualization layer. Here, data processing and analytics tools are employed to extract actionable insights from the collected data, aiding in clinical decision-making and patient care.
- The fifth layer of IoMT architecture, similar to IoT's application/integration layer, provides the business functionality by integrating applications and platforms with the IoMT infrastructure. This integration enables the utilization of collected data to enhance healthcare processes, facilitate informed decision-making, and deliver personalized patient services.
- Lastly, IoMT, like IoT, encompasses a sixth layer dedicated to security and management. This layer ensures the security and proper management of the entire IoMT infrastructure, safeguarding sensitive patient data and devices against external threats and ensuring the system's smooth operation and performance·

As Figure 1.2 shows, IoMT architecture provides a structured framework for designing, implementing, and managing IoMT systems, leveraging connected devices and data to revolutionize healthcare delivery. Understanding and coordinating the various layers of the architecture are essential for developing effective and secure IoMT solutions tailored to the unique needs of healthcare environments [16].

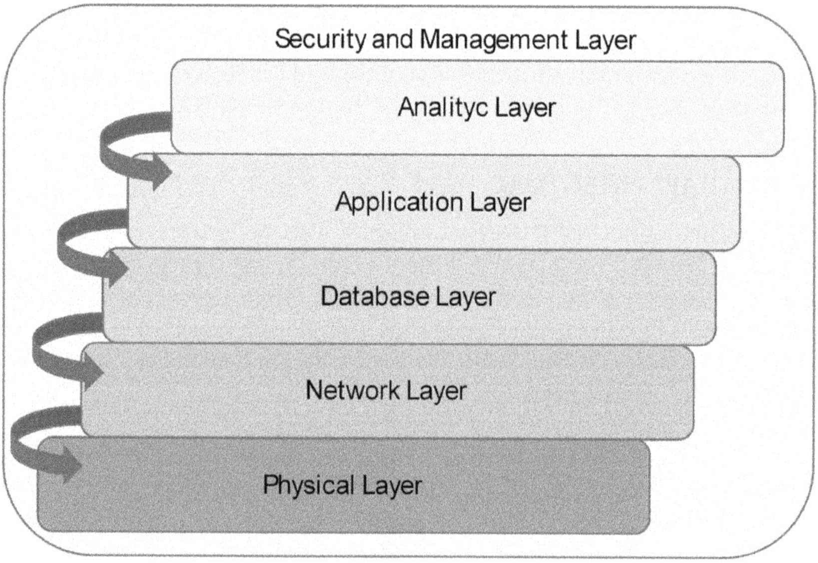

FIGURE 1.2 IoMT architecture.

1.3.1 IoMT Sensing Systems

The sensing systems for IoMT are sensors that measure variables from the persons monitored in their environment in order to provide accurate data about their health status. The used sensors have a huge variation and can be classified based on different aspects. Regarding the location of sensors, these can be wearable or non-wearable.

On the one hand, wearable sensors, generally characterized by their small size and high robustness, are placed close to the monitored person, mostly in bracelets, bands, or smartwatches. These sensors might measure aspects such as movement, breathing, heart rate, sweating, body temperature, or oxygen saturation, among others. Nonetheless, another type of wearable sensor includes printed sensors, which can be embedded directly in the skin or in clothes. A third type of wearable sensor, considered an invasive sensor, is located inside the monitored people for measuring blood, generally for glucose monitoring. These are only used in chronic patient monitoring.

On the other hand, non-wearable sensors are placed in the area in which the monitored person is located. These are generally used for monitoring the indoor environment in which the monitored person is located, generally their house or the hospital. Focusing on house monitoring, these sensors monitor the environmental variables, such as temperature, humidity, sound, and air quality, but they can also monitor the person themselves with the presence of sensors. Meanwhile, the sensors in the hospitals for IoMT are more specific and might be monitoring the operation of medical devices and their surroundings, such as the bed, intravenous drip, or oxygen concentrator. A summary of different sensors and their classification are included in Figure 1.3.

1.3.2 IoMT Communication Technologies

The following section describes different types of communications and technologies. Its characteristics are described (distance, bitrate, license, indoor/outdoor,

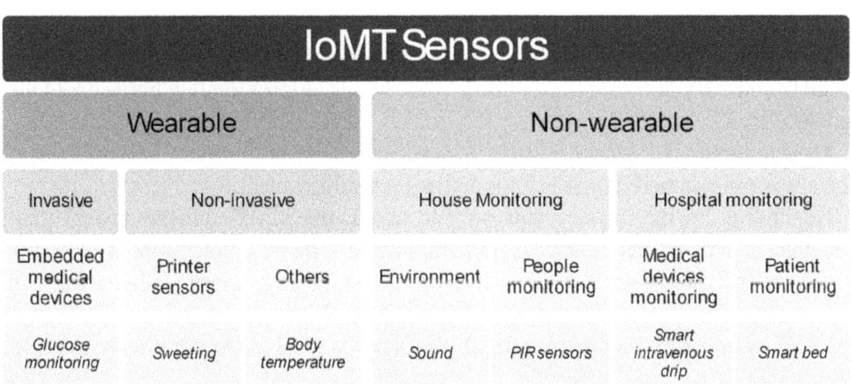

FIGURE 1.3 Classification of sensors on IoMT according to their location and purpose.

TABLE 1.1
Summary of Communication Technologies Which Can Be Used for IoMT

Technologies	Distance	Bitrate	License	Energy consumption
IEEE 802.15.4	10–75 m	20–250 kbps	Licensed/ Unlicensed	−25 dBm/−0 dBm
IEEE 802.11n	70 m/ 250 m	600 Mbps	Unlicensed	
IEEE 802.11ac wave 2	70 m/ 250 m	7,000 Mbps	Unlicensed	
Bluetooth 2.0	10 m	2.1 Mbps	Unlicensed	Not specified
Bluetooth 3.0	10 m	24 Mbps	Unlicensed	Not specified
Bluetooth 5.0	350 m	1–2–3 Mbps	Unlicensed	1–100 mW
ANT+	100 m/20 m	1 Mbps	Unlicensed	–
RuBee	30 m	1,024 bps	Licensed	–
Insteon	–	2,880 bps	Unlicensed	–
Z-Wave	30 m	9.6/40 kbps	Licensed/ Unlicensed	Low
IEEE 802.16e (WiMAX)	50 km	15– 90 Mbps	Licensed	
5G	300 km	10–50 Gb/s	Both	
LoRa	22 km	290 bps to 50 kbps	Unlicensed	

energy consumption, and capability). These characteristics are specific to each type of technology and allow us to understand the transmission and reception of data (see Table 1.1). Examples of Wi-Fi, Bluetooth, 5G, and LoRa networks, among others, are shown.

In general, most technologies cover distances in meters; however, others cover kilometers (WiMAX, 5G, and LoRa). In addition, there are differences in the frequency bands used by each type of communication. It should be noted that the most used frequency is generally 2.4 GHz. However, others, such as LoRa, use 868 and 900 MHz. 5G operates in low bands (around 600 MHz to 1 GHz), mid bands (between 1.8 GHz and 2.6 GHz), and high or mm Wave bands (approximately between 24 GHz and 40 GHz).

Most technologies do not require licenses and cover both indoor and outdoor use. The energy consumed depends a lot on the technology used.

Depending on the devices you want to use in the IoMT and the system that is designed, it will be necessary to implement one type of connection. It is possible to use several kinds simultaneously, always considering, among other things, the distance and data transmission speed. Commonly, the health domain uses Wi-Fi and 802.15.4 technology. Meanwhile, IEEE 802.11ah is used in the healthcare domain.

1.3.3 IoMT and Energy-Related Issues

The IoMT faces energy constraints across various aspects of its operation. Key challenges include ensuring the power efficiency of devices, optimizing wireless communication, managing data processing and storage, promoting sustainability in healthcare infrastructure, and complying with regulatory standards [17].

Device power efficiency is crucial to extend battery life and reduce the need for frequent recharging or replacement. This involves designing devices with low-power components and implementing energy-saving modes. Wireless communication, essential for transmitting health data, consumes energy, particularly in scenarios with high transmission rates. So, the optimization of communication protocols and frequencies can alleviate this constraint.

On the other hand, data processing and storage tasks, such as real-time monitoring and predictive analytics, require computational resources that consume energy. Energy-efficient algorithms, edge computing, and cloud optimization strategies can mitigate this problem. Sustainable practices in building and maintaining IoMT infrastructure, including data centers and networking equipment, are essential for reducing energy consumption and environmental impact.

Compliance with energy efficiency standards and environmental regulations promotes responsible energy consumption and environmental stewardship within the IoMT ecosystem. By prioritizing energy efficiency, adopting sustainable technologies, and adhering to regulatory standards, the IoMT industry can address energy constraints while advancing healthcare innovation and improving patient outcomes.

1.3.4 IoMT and AI

AI also has a significant role in the IoMT and is involved in different parts of the IoMT systems. We can distinguish two main uses of AI: (a) for data management and detection of abnormal situations and for (b) prediction of abnormal situations in the future given the current data. There might be a third use of AI to automatically react, including actuators, when an abnormal situation is detected. Nevertheless, the current regulations in several countries do not allow this use.

AI comprises a large number of tools and algorithms which are characterized by different features and, therefore, applied for different purposes. In Figure 1.4, we have shown the classification of AI.

According to the process followed by ML to learn from data, there are three types of ML: supervised, unsupervised, and reinforcement learning. Supervised ML is mainly used to generate classification and regression models based on a subset of previously labeled data. Meanwhile, unsupervised ML is generally used for clustering purposes and uses data which has not been labeled. Finally, reinforced learning is aimed at evaluating the better action given a series of parameters and the previous actions. This is not necessarily applied for triggering actuators, it can also be applied to generate alarms and detect abnormal situations.

Deep learning can also be divided into generative, discriminative, and hybrid techniques. Based on unsupervised methods, generative deep learning has multiple

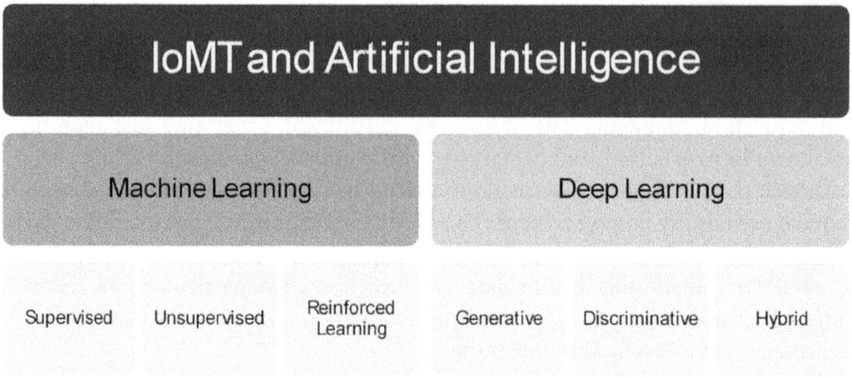

FIGURE 1.4 Classification of artificial intelligence for IoMT.

layers from the input layer to the output layer, acting as a black box, and is generally used to discover high-order correlation properties of a given data. Discriminative deep learning is based on supervised methods and is generally used to provide a discriminative function for pattern classification.

1.3.5 Security in IoMT

The security requirements for IoMT systems are multifaceted and crucial for ensuring the integrity and confidentiality of medical data in digital healthcare systems. Recognizing the vulnerability of IoMT devices to cyber threats, the text emphasizes the strategic implementation of security measures across the network infrastructure. Compliance with the CIAAA principle (confidentiality [C], integrity [I], availability [A] of data, accountability [A] and authenticity [A]) serves as the cornerstone for addressing security concerns within IoMT ecosystems [18]:

- Confidentiality is paramount in protecting sensitive medical information shared between patients and healthcare providers. Measures such as network access control and data encryption are essential for safeguarding against unauthorized access and eavesdropping attempts. Privacy regulations like General Data Protection Regulation (GDPR) [19] and Health Insurance Portability and Accountability Act (HIPAA) [20] further underscore the importance of protecting patients' personal health information from unlawful disclosure or exploitation, ensuring compliance and maintaining trust in IoMT systems.
- Data integrity is crucial for preserving the accuracy and reliability of patient data during transmission and storage. Healthcare organizations prioritize data integrity to safeguard critical information related to diagnoses, treatments, and health statuses, bolstering trust in IoMT systems.
- Availability ensures continuous access to healthcare services and data, essential for monitoring patients' health statuses. Robust measures against

Denial-of-Service (DoS) and Distributed Denial-of-Service (DDoS) attacks are necessary to uphold availability and ensure uninterrupted healthcare services.
- Non-repudiation enhances accountability within IoMT systems by holding authorized users responsible for their actions, preventing the denial of system activities, and enhancing trust and integrity in system operations.
- Authentication mechanisms verify user identities and authenticate transmitted data, ensuring the authenticity and integrity of information exchanged within IoMT networks. Lightweight authentication algorithms address resource constraints in IoMT devices, facilitating secure data exchange.
- Authorization mechanisms restrict access to sensitive medical data, mitigating the risk of unauthorized access and safeguarding patient privacy. Anonymity preserves patient and physician identities during system interactions, shielding them from passive observation and unauthorized disclosure, fostering trust and confidentiality in healthcare communications within IoMT ecosystems.

Compliance with these security requirements is imperative for fortifying IoMT networks' security posture and protecting the integrity and confidentiality of patient data in digital healthcare environments [21]. Figure 1.5 shows a summary of the main vulnerabilities in IoMT and which mechanisms could be used to guarantee the total safety of a system with medical purposes.

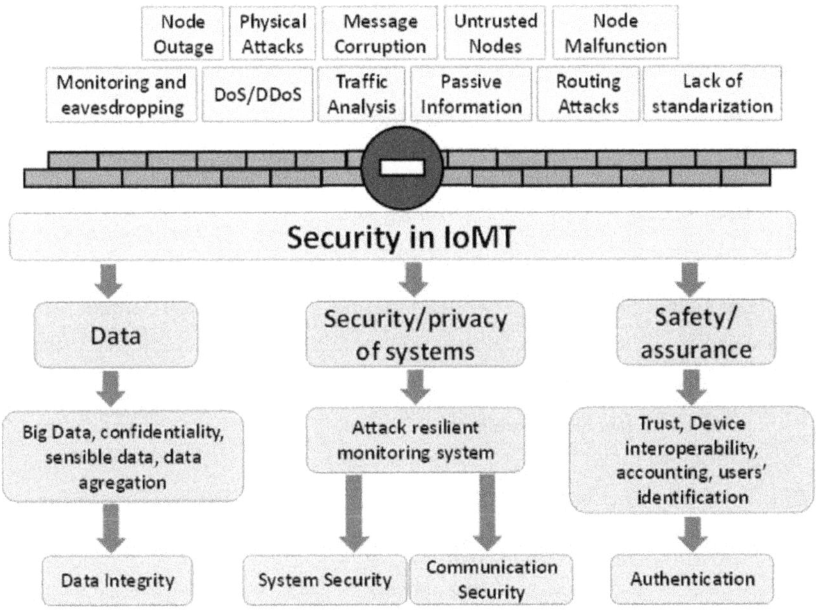

FIGURE 1.5 Vulnerabilities in IoMT and how to solve them.

1.3.6 Data Management in IoMT

The data management in IoMT is critical for different reasons. First of all, the early detection of alarms is vital to enhance patient empowerment. Moreover, adequate data management is crucial to maximizing energy efficiency, thus reducing required batteries and extending the node lifetime. For those purposes, data management can be conducted at different levels in the IoMT architecture (see Figure 1.6). It is possible to distinguish three main levels of data management: edge computing, fog computing, and cloud computing.

In edge computing, data is managed in the node itself. In the node, data from different connected sensors can be analyzed to identify abnormal situations and react to these alterations. The tools used for analyzing data depend on the node computational capacity and are generally limited to applying rules of predefined machine learning models trained in computers.

Fog computing involves the combination of data from multiple nodes and the network at a higher level. This action is conducted by a device with computing capability located between the node and the cloud. These devices have higher computation capacity than the node and can compute more complex models such as unsupervised machine learning. Beyond the actions described in edge computing, data fusion and optimization of energy in the network are some of the common actions in fog computing. The actions taken can be applied directly to the computing devices or to nodes.

Finally, cloud computing is performed by a server in the cloud. In this server, data from the network can be combined with data from external sources. In cloud

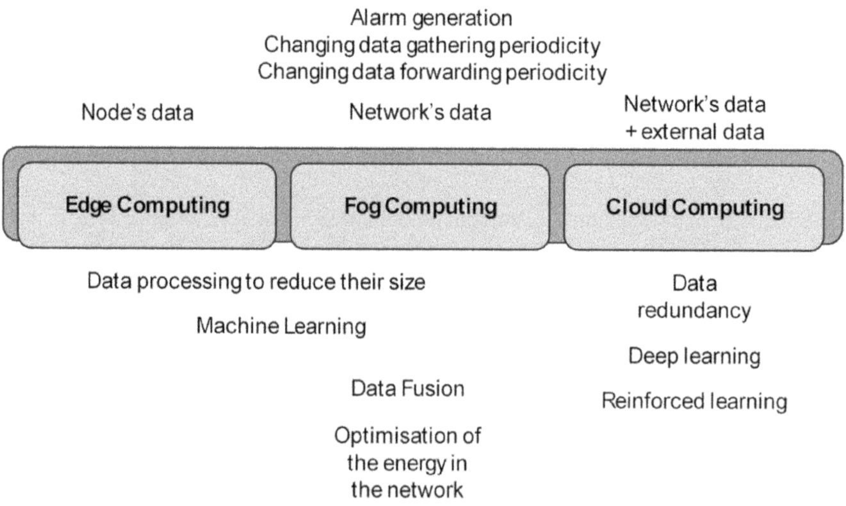

FIGURE 1.6 Details of different types of computing included in the IoMT networks.

computing, the integration of experts can be considered to include reinforced learning. Moreover, the higher computation capacity of servers allows for deep learning.

1.4 ANALYSIS

In this section, we present the results of a specific case of use. We include data from an IoMT system for sleep monitoring of a patient with asthma. There is clear evidence that indicates that asthma and apnea are closely related [22]. Moreover, asthma patients tend to cough at night, especially when the allergens are present in the environment. Different pollutants might have a diverse presence in indoor and outdoor environments, and monitoring systems can provide updated information on them [23].

The proposed system comprises a microphone embedded in a pillow, as proposed in Ref. [24]. The system uses edge computing to determine if data corresponds to regular noise while sleeping or if there is a sound that needs to be verified. To do this, a simple threshold is applied to determine the maximum sound in 15 seconds of recording. A series of sounds are presented in Figure 1.7. According to the gathered data, we have established a threshold value of 60 dB. The data gathered during normal breath does not exceed 45 dB at any moment, and the average sound is 36 dB. Nonetheless, breath with nasal congestion (see Figure 1.7a) and breath through the mouth (see Figure 1.7b) have peak values of 54–58 dB and an erratic trend with averaged values of about 40 dB and minimum values of 30 and 31 dB.

All records, including peak values above 60 dB, are supposed to include sounds that need to be characterized. In the tests, we included coughing, coughing lightly, sneezing, yawning, snoring, and snoring before apnea as a sound during the night. These sounds will be identified by supervised machine learning algorithms applied to the gateway as fog computing. The sounds include cough, coughing lightly, and sneezing, which are generally produced when the patient is exposed to allergens.

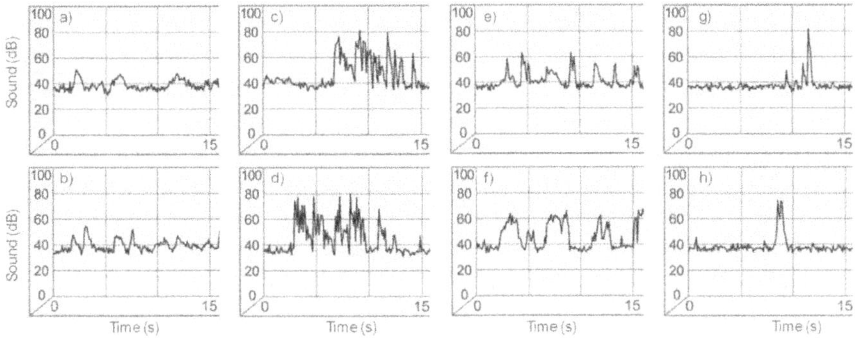

FIGURE 1.7 Sound to test the system. (a) Breath with nasal congestion. (b) Breath through the mouth. (c) Cough. (d) Cough lightly. (e) Snore. (f) Snore before apnea. (g) Sneeze. (h) Yawn.

Cough and cough lightly (see Figure 1.7c and d) are characterized by peak values of 80 ± 1 dB and average values of 45 ± 2 dB.

Two records of obstructive apnea are included. The first record consists of regular snoring (see Figure 1.7e), while the second is the sound preceding an apnea (see Figure 1.7f). The main difference is not in the maxim value, which is similar (67.8 and 67.6 dB). In this case, the shape of the curve and the average value (41.4 and 46.1 dB) are determinants for the correct classification.

Yawning (see Figure 1.7h) is an additional sound that can be easily confused with sneezing (see Figure 1.7g) due to its acute angle in the peak. It must be noted that the record in which the patient has sneezed is the one with the highest sound value (82.4 dB), and the yawning record is the one with the lowest peak value (74.2 dB). These records have low average values (37.5 and 38.2 dB) since sound is produced only in a short period of time, generally less than 1 second.

After classifying the sound, the system tags the data. If data corresponds to an extreme situation, such as stopping breathing due to apnea, and the situation is not solved in two records (30 seconds), then a sound is emitted to wake up the patient. At the end of the night, all the records are sent to the server, where reinforced machine learning is applied based on medical input.

1.5 CONCLUSIONS

The IoMT is the use of IoT for medical purposes with the main aim of improving patient empowerment, having reliable data about patient status, and improving the provided medical services. The IoMT systems are composed of many elements, among which we can highlight the sensing systems, communication technologies, and nodes with diverse computational capacities. The data gathered by the sensor nodes can be managed at different levels, including edge computing, fog computing, and cloud computing by means of artificial intelligence. Thus, the energy efficiency can be improved. Other critical aspects of the correct operation of IoMT systems are security and data formats. These aspects ensure that health providers can use the data.

In this chapter, we have presented a general introduction to the different elements of the IoMT systems and an example of an IoMT system. First of all, different elements of the IoMT architecture have been defined, and examples have been provided. Then, in the results, we analyzed how different sounds can be used to classify different sleep disorders, such as coughing, snoring, or breathing through the mouth, among others. Sounds were collected overnight while a patient with asthma was asleep. The records used have a duration of 15 seconds. The obtained data is compared to differentiate the origin of recorded sounds by assessing the average and maximum sound values. In addition, for some sounds, the shape of the curve is necessary to clearly identify the origin of the sound. Thus, a combination of supervised machine learning in edge computing and reinforced learning in cloud computing has been proposed.

In the following chapters, each of these elements will be analyzed in detail, deepening in the particularities and limitations. Moreover, study cases and the different uses of IoMT are analyzed to provide a comprehensive vision of the current status of IoMT and its potential benefits for society.

REFERENCES:

1. Kamruzzaman, M. M., Alrashdi, I., & Alqazzaz, A. (2022). New opportunities, challenges, and applications of edge-AI for connected healthcare in internet of medical things for smart cities. *Journal of Healthcare Engineering*, 2022, 2950699. https://doi.org/10.1155/2022/2950699
2. Dwivedi, R., Mehrotra, D., & Chandra, S. (2022). Potential of Internet of Medical Things (IoMT) applications in building a smart healthcare system: A systematic review. *Journal of Oral Biology and Craniofacial Research*, 12(2), 302–318.
3. Sun, H., De Florio, V., Gui, N., & Blondia, C. (2009, April). Promises and challenges of ambient assisted living systems. In *2009 Sixth International Conference on Information Technology: New Generations* (pp. 1201–1207). IEEE.
4. Ahmed, S., Naga Srinivasu, P., Alhumam, A., & Alarfaj, M. (2022). AAL and internet of medical things for monitoring type-2 diabetic patients. *Diagnostics*, 12(11), 2739.
5. Rajawat, A. S., Goyal, S. B., Bedi, P., Jan, T., Whaiduzzaman, M., & Prasad, M. (2023). Quantum machine learning for security assessment in the Internet of Medical Things (IoMT). *Future Internet*, 15(8), 271.
6. Gupta, D., Bhatia, M. P. S., & Kumar, A. (2021). Resolving data overload and latency issues in multivariate time-series IoMT data for mental health monitoring. *IEEE Sensors Journal*, 21(22), 25421–25428.
7. Das, J., Do, Q. T., Friedman, J., & McKenzie, D. (2009). Mental health patterns and consequences: Results from survey data in five developing countries. *The World Bank Economic Review*, 23(1), 31–55.
8. Razdan, S., & Sharma, S. (2022). Internet of Medical Things (IoMT): Overview, emerging technologies, and case studies. *IETE Technical Review*, 39(4), 775-788.
9. World Wide Science Web. Available at: https://worldwidescience.org/wws/desktop/en/results.html. Last access (05/04/2024).
10. Hernandez-Jaimes, M. L., Martinez-Cruz, A., Ramírez-Gutiérrez, K. A., & Feregrino-Uribe, C. (2023). Artificial intelligence for IoMT security: A review of intrusion detection systems, attacks, datasets and Cloud-Fog-Edge architectures. *Internet of Things*, 23, 100887.
11. Mahmood, M., Khan, M. I., Hussain, H., Khan, I., Rahman, S., Shabir, M., & Niazi, B. (2023). *Improving Security Architecture of Internet of Medical Things: A Systematic Literature Review*. IEEE Access.
12. Bhushan, B., Kumar, A., Agarwal, A. K., Kumar, A., Bhattacharya, P., & Kumar, A. (2023). Towards a secure and sustainable Internet of Medical Things (IoMT): Requirements, design challenges, security techniques, and future trends. *Sustainability*, 15(7), 6177.
13. Ghubaish, A., Salman, T., Zolanvari, M., Unal, D., Al-Ali, A., & Jain, R. (2020). Recent advances in the Internet-of-Medical-Things (IoMT) systems security. *IEEE Internet of Things Journal*, 8(11), 8707–8718.
14. Vishnu, S., Ramson, S. J., & Jegan, R. (2020, March). Internet of Medical Things (IoMT)-An overview. In *2020 5th International Conference on Devices, Circuits and Systems (ICDCS)* (pp. 101–104). IEEE.
15. Manickam, P., Mariappan, S. A., Murugesan, S. M., Hansda, S., Kaushik, A., Shinde, R., & Thipperudraswamy, S. P. (2022). Artificial Intelligence (AI) and Internet of Medical Things (IoMT) assisted biomedical systems for intelligent healthcare. *Biosensors*, 12(8), 562.

16. Ashfaq, Z., Rafay, A., Mumtaz, R., Zaidi, S. M. H., Saleem, H., Zaidi, S. A. R., ... & Haque, A. (2022). A review of enabling technologies for Internet of Medical Things (IoMT) Ecosystem. *Ain Shams Engineering Journal*, 13(4), 101660.
17. 6 IoT Architecture Layers and Components Explained. Available at: https://www.techtarget.com/iotagenda/tip/A-comprehensive-view-of-the-4-IoT-architecture-layers. Last access (22/04/2024).
18. Saba, T., Haseeb, K., Ahmed, I., & Rehman, A. (2020). Secure and energy-efficient framework using internet of medical things for e-healthcare. *Journal of Infection and Public Health*, 13(10), 1567–1575.
19. Kaur, G., Habibi Lashkari, Z., Habibi Lashkari, A., Kaur, G., Habibi Lashkari, Z., & Habibi Lashkari, A. (2021). Introduction to cybersecurity. In *Understanding Cybersecurity Management in FinTech: Challenges, Strategies, and Trends* (pp. 17–34). Springer.
20. GDPR vs. HIPAA: Differences and Compliance. Available at: https://secureprivacy.ai/blog/gdpr-hipaa-similarities-differences-health-data-compliance. Last access (22/04/2024).
21. Pear, R. (2017). White House proposes new rules to steady insurance markets under health law. *International New York Times*.
22. Fiaidhi, J., & Mohammed, S. (2019). Security and vulnerability of extreme automation systems: The IoMT and IoA case studies. *IT Professional*, 21(4), 48–55.
23. Teodorescu, M., Barnet, J. H., Hagen, E. W., Palta, M., Young, T. B., & Peppard, P. E. (2015). Association between asthma and risk of developing obstructive sleep apnea. *JAMA*, 313(2), 156–164.
24. Wang, J., Viciano-Tudela, S., Parra, L., Lacuesta, R., & Lloret, J. (2023). Evaluation of suitability of low-cost gas sensors for monitoring indoor and outdoor urban areas. *IEEE Sensors Journal*, 23, 20968–20975.
25. Veiga, A., Garcia, L., Parra, L., Lloret, J., & Augele, V. (2018, April). An IoT-based smart pillow for sleep quality monitoring in AAL environments. In *2018 Third International Conference on Fog and Mobile Edge Computing (FMEC)* (pp. 175–180). IEEE.

2 Optimizing Smart Hospitals with IoMT

A Deep Dive into the Next-Generation Paradigm for Digital Healthcare

Maharaja Muthuvairam Subbulakshmi, Pradeep Kumar Sriram, Jeyakanthan Jeyaraman, and Gomathinayagam Subramanian

2.1 INTRODUCTION

Modern healthcare has experienced a remarkable transformation due to the development of advanced diagnostic systems. The recent trend of Artificial Intelligence (AI) and Machine Learning (ML) is rapidly being applied to IoMT (Internet of Medical Things) through medical devices, revolutionizing the healthcare sector. Therefore, Healthcare 4.0 signifies a modern breakthrough in integrating AI with IoMT for health management systems. This innovative approach enables healthcare professionals to connect with and monitor medical devices via the Internet. Consequently, IoMT provides strong support for robust healthcare management, facilitating cost-effectiveness, faster real-time transmission, and personalized patient care with timely interventions [1]. To grasp the latest advancements in IoMT, it is essential to trace back the development chronology of Internet of Things (IoT). IoTs are prominently paired with electronic devices and sensors with innovative real-time applications in diverse industrial sectors. The nodes of the Internet are connected across multiple domains and also interconnect individuals via smart gadgets. The progress of IoT has led to impressive achievements in establishing smart classes, smart homes, smart transport, and smart cities. Among these accomplishments, the medical system has not been an exception. The IoT system that deeply integrates diagnostic and prognostic medical systems, providing forecasted outcomes, is termed IoMT. In recent times, the IoMT has emerged as a novel platform in healthcare, assisting professionals in providing effective treatment. The IoMT acts as a junction for objects and medical systems, particularly in MRI, CT, and other sophisticated clinical equipment [2]. To gain preliminary insights into the operational mechanism of an IoMT framework,

DOI: 10.1201/9781003476344-2

it is essential to understand the adoption of its architectures. The COVID-19 outbreak catalyzed the shift toward digitalized healthcare services. The IoMT enabled the remote monitoring of the outbreak along with various other healthcare services. The IoMT-operated sensors incorporated in wearable devices provide a non-invasive method for monitoring critical parameters of the body's organs [3]. The implementation of IoMT systems in the various modern healthcare services, including diagnosis, remote monitoring, and resource allocation, has greatly enabled the understanding and facilitates in the improvement of existing facilities. AI–ML algorithms incorporated into IoMT systems enhance the effective treatment protocols for improved patient care. The remote monitoring sensors on the IoMT systems can effectively detect the spread of disease during a pandemic situation. The IoMT can be an analytic tool for analyzing data like disease transmission trends and patterns. The IoMT system can cluster semistructured, unstructured, or structured data from enormous volumes of Zettabytes (ZB) of data to manageable chunks of terabytes (TB) of data obtained from assorted origins. These systems can synergize with GPS (Global Positioning Systems) supporting 4G, 5G, and 6G bandwidth technologies for the containment of disease monitoring [4]. In 2020, over 5.2 billion of the global population opted for mobile services, which steadily climbed to 5.7 billion in 2025, which is more than 70% of the global population. Hence, the IoT on smartphones and wearable gadgets adopted IoMT, which was constructed to alert the outbreaks and self-care practices for handling infectious diseases. Although the global population depends upon vaccination, the IoMT systems supporting vaccination programs ought to provide functionalities of scalability and data privacy. This should also extend the capabilities of live updates regarding the supply chain of the vaccines and rapid reports along with real-time decision-making protocols [5]. The elevation of IoMT has potentially been achieved with the big data clustering along with wireless technologies, with efficiency and accessibility being shifted to next-generation smart healthcare systems. This chapter explores and illustrates the revolution of the architectural framework and the technology enabling IoMT devices in smart healthcare.

2.2 INTERNET OF MEDICAL THINGS (IOMT)

The IoMT is a confederation of biomedical devices for healthcare surveillance with futuristic network architectures. Medical support personnel and surgeons have to conduct routine rounds on a shift basis to monitor patients' health status kept for observation. However, the IoMT implementation potentially puts forward the foundations for adaptive systems with reliability, offering personalized assistance with real-time patient surveillance computed with smart sensing and continued rigorous diagnosis. In 2018, the market level of IoMT was calculated at 44.50 billion dollars globally, and the projection has touched 254.20 billion dollars in the 2025–2026 interim period and is calculated to grow at a compound annual growth rate (CAGR) scaling up of 24.6%. The feature of an IoMT system is usually confined to an endpoint within the device, providing a gateway for autonomous connection to the cloud. The biosensors equipped with transmitters like NB-IoT (narrowband IoT) and ZigBee will actively link to the router [6]. The PHI (personal health information) of the patients were digitalized to EHRs (electronic health records) enabling higher accuracy for screening. The deep learning (DL) algorithm of the IoMT medical devices enhances CAD (computer-aided diagnosis) by calibrating over 80% with sensitivity and accuracy. The IoMT incorporates AI-computerized visualization technologies like medical imaging and processing. Recently, a CVT (computer vision technique) was incorporated with a CNN-ML (convolutional neural network–machine learning) system and was used to detect liver cancer lesions, proceeding with AI imaging. It is also a diagnostic tool. The 5G technology has also elevated modern medical systems with advancements in communication, providing large-scale connectivity and extending to virtual networks. Hence, the 5G network has extended the applicability of remote patient monitoring (RPM) through ultrafast, high-bandwidth connections which offer stability, real-time data transmission, and reduced latency [7].

2.3 ARCHITECTURAL FRAMEWORK OF IOMT

The architectural framework of IoMT extensively proposes the architectures of IoTs along with the web of things, sensor-based network, and built-in M2M (machine-to-machine) settings. Predominantly, the IoMT system was built with several phases of equilibrium, like data collection, management, and service provider. Several parameters like body temperature, ECG (electrocardiogram), blood pressure, and glucose level were detected and transferred via medical sensors from a data collection layer. The fog layer acts as an interface between the medical data collection and the cloud services. This layer was developed to handle multiple local servers that are connected via the thinly spread-out fog network. The clustered medical data was preprocessed by edge servers and allocated storage for each data on the management layer. This framework computes cloud data and big data for effective analysis and processing of data storage. In addition, healthcare professionals administer and supervise the medical services layer, ensuring only authorized access to the entire IoMT network and maintaining data privacy [8]. These standard layers were built to enhance the robust nature of the IoMT architecture. Some advancements in IoMT architecture include PUF (physically unclonable function) devices and SDN (software-defined networking) tabulated in Table 2.1 and picturized in Figure 2.1. These innovations aim to improve data privacy employed in an IoMT network through various factors, such as identifying vulnerabilities or miscreants in the system, hardware tampering, device authentication, and securing communication protocols [9].

2.4 INCORPORATION OF IOMT IN HEALTHCARE SERVICES

Sensors are the core of IoMT, broadly sensing various physiological indicators like glucose level, heart rate, oxygen saturation, temperature, blood pressure, light intensity, gravity, velocity, noise levels, and humidity. Wearable sensors can readily detect heart rate through the wristband, while the fixed device measures blood oxygen saturation levels. These sensors can also be fixed on medical examination instruments, enhancing diagnosis and screening the degree of prognosis. Recent advancements indicate that IoMT devices are outperforming traditional approaches

TABLE 2.1
Major Features Streaming on IoMT-Enabled Devices

Feature	Criteria
Signal quality	The 5G communication technologies enable high-quality signal transmission
Usability	In wearable devices, the sensors are non-instructive, lightweight and easy to use
Sensing technology	The architecture includes PUF (physically unclonable function) devices and SDN (software-defined networking)
Reliability	Highly capable of providing accurate and reliable pulse rate readings
Compatibility	Compatible with the intended medical instruments or systems

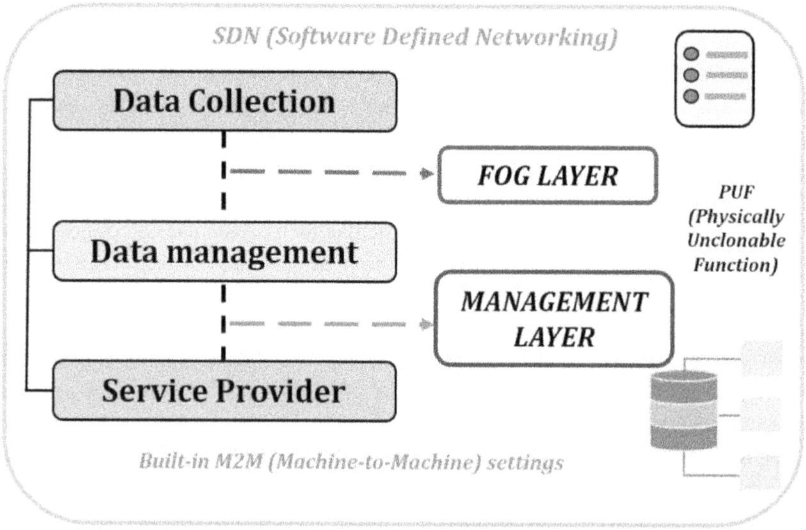

FIGURE 2.1 A concise representation of built-in phases of the IoMT system.

of manual microscopic counting with regard to analyzing whole blood cell counting [10]. In 2021, an applied IoMT device was adopted on a CT instrument to effectively perform the scanning process with higher efficiency. In this context, the accuracy and real-time capability of the IoMT dominate traditional medical examination [11]. The IoMT-body detectors examine the behavior of the human body categorizing emotions, movements, expressions, and postures. On the other hand, environmental sensing visible light cameras, infrared detectors, and indoor radars have also been advanced with ML algorithms. This IoMT surveillance system has been coupled with CVA (computer vision algorithms), assisting in tracking the environmental trajectories [12]. Especially, the latest CVT on the IoMT devices enables real-time analysis of planning strictly segmented zones in healthcare centers, warning people of

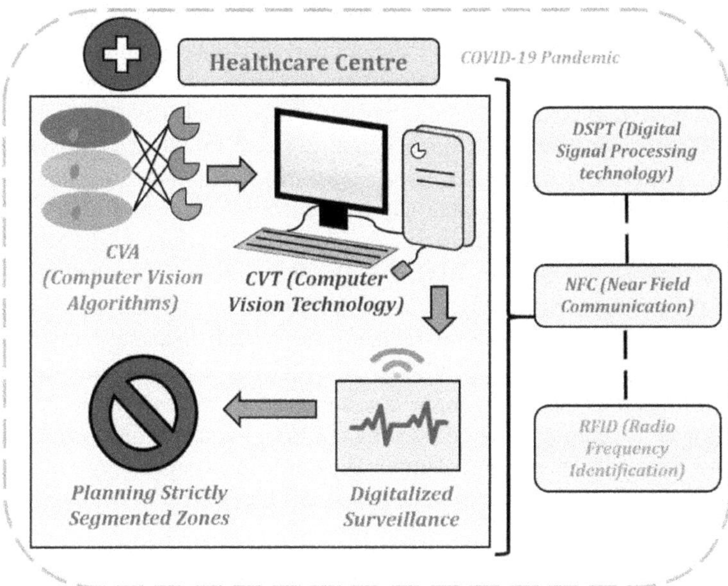

FIGURE 2.2 A graphical representation of the IoMT surveillance system during the COVID-19 pandemic.

unauthorized entry to avoid the spread of nosocomial infections. The infrared detectors sense human activity and detect body temperature, which was highly utilized during the COVID-19 pandemic period [13]. The installation of indoor radars like laser radar, ultrasound radar, and millimeter-wave radar in hospitals, rehabilitation centers, and nursing homes enables monitoring activity and realizing fall detection. In real time, applied indoor radar was designed as a disinfectant robot that automatically recognizes and disinfects risk areas, avoiding human infection [14]. The applied RFID (radio-frequency identification) and NFC (near field communication) technologies incorporated the components for developing smart hospitals, as demonstrated in Figure 2.2. The IoMT devices upgraded on ambulances provide improved patient care and emergency treatment en route using quick e-healthcare services. Hence, medical devices upgraded with IoMT systems have transformed the landscape of healthcare services, which once primarily relied on traditional assets [15].

2.5 IOMT DEVICES TRANSFORMING SMART HOSPITALS

The concept of smart hospitals spawned in the 1980s and has remained theoretical for the past 20 years or so. But with the advent of IoMT systems in hospitals, smart hospitals have come much closer to reality. A smart hospital was first described or defined as a healthcare-providing institution that focuses on applying procedures and protocols that can lead to improved asset management, resulting in reduced medical care provision expenditure and a decrease in patient-related accidents. In the current era of IoMT devices and the widespread availability of wearable sensor devices, this definition has greatly changed. At present, a smart hospital can support high levels of automation in functioning, boost productivity, and reduce errors in patient diagnosis and prognosis. All these aims can thus be achieved relatively easily, with the deployment of AI and other knowledge management systems [16]. With the arrival of innovative technologies, such as smartphones, wearable health monitors, smart sensors, and inexpensive data storage solutions, the recording and analytics of biomedical data have become much more feasible compared to older days. Multi-billion-dollar business conglomerates such as IBM, Google, and Siemens have also focused their research and development ventures toward the development of smart hospitals since it is a viable business initiative for reducing the overall financial burden imposed upon healthcare providers [17]. In addition, the services or features that can be found in smart hospitals include short-range communications to track services, facilitated by high-speed 5G communication networks, RFID, barcodes, QR (quick response) codes, and GPS [18]. Therefore, the application of IoMT systems looks highly promising to transform our current hospitals into smart hospitals.

2.6 ROLE OF IOMT IN COVID-19 MANAGEMENT

The outbreak of COVID-19 acted as a catalyst for medical instruments to adopt IoMTs. The IoMT leverages cloud computing to incorporate healthcare devices and equipment. The IoMT was crucial in tracing and monitoring the COVID-19 outbreak, assisting healthcare professionals in managing the disease effectively. It also facilitated immediate diagnostic tests, accurately leading to the treatment and monitoring of physiological conditions. The IoMT's phenomenal growth encouraged DSPT (digital signal processing technologies) to embed with medical devices. Hence, the advancement helped healthcare professionals manage medical data to receive alerts on critical scenarios and generate real-time solutions. The IoMT conducted contact tracing, which secured a key role in the pandemic, to generate immediate warnings to the people who were in contact with infected individuals. Compared to traditional contact tracking like manual recording, the employment of Wi-Fi and Bluetooth proved to be a faster approach with accurate results. Due to the higher rate of contagiousness of the virus, the IoMT devices were used for sensing body temperatures to detect affected patients [19]. The IoMT real-time tracking devices, like wearable bands and disinfectant devices, were implemented for the effective management of the pandemic. The mass collection of medical data has also been crucial for predicting or preventing future outbreaks. The collaboration of EHRs and IoMT data-collecting devices observed and obtained the COVID-19 health-related data, which was clustered and communicated to servers with secured authentication [20]. The emergence of disruptive innovations like AI, 5G networks, and cloud computing platforms has coordinately built a framework for managing the COVID-19 pandemic. Table 2.2 illustrates the key aspects that assisted doctors in carrying out effective diagnoses and speeding up decisions to take care of patients in home quarantine or to treat the patient in a hospital, along with the appropriate resources. Hence, the implementation of the IoMT smart framework has boosted

TABLE 2.2
Illustrating the Key Aspectsof IoMT on the COVID-19 Outbreak

Key Aspect	Description
Cloud computing	Leveraging cloud computing connected to servers, the IoMT systems monitored the outbreaks
Contact tracking	Facilitated accurate and faster tracking through DSPT (digital signal processing technology)
Sensing body temperature	IoMT instrument detects elevated body temperatures and supported home quarantine treatment decisions
Real-time monitoring	Wearable bands and smart gadgets like disinfectant devices contributed effective disease management
Smart IoMT framework	Incorporating DMS (digital monitoring system) and cloud computing architectures potentially managed the outbreak

the diagnosis and treatment and facilitated network services through DMS (Digital Monitoring System), authorized cloud computing, data analytics tools, and sensing and scanning tools [21].

2.7 IOMT IN DRUG DEVELOPMENT AND PHARMACEUTICALS

The COVID-19 outbreak between 2020 and 2022 revealed the immediate need for new drugs that can be used to combat emerging viral and bacterial infections. The arrival of IoMT systems in the market has made it possible to increase the rate of discovery of new drugs and their subsequent development. To build a foundation for using IoMTs in drug discovery, a framework has already been proposed. However, these technologies remain in the future, while research is also taking place. This proposed framework, which has been exclusively framed for identifying novel antiviral drugs, involves the identification of the virus, predicting feasible viral antigens, and animal model immunization, which ultimately leads to the development of a novel vaccine or drug [22]. This framework not only utilizes IoMT devices to generate the data but also proposes to employ computationally intelligent algorithms such as ML, DL, and edge computing (EC) to process the generated data. Therefore, the AI revolution in IoMT devices can potentially help pharmaceutical companies and research institutes to maximize their efficiency in producing large quantities of life-saving vaccines, without compromising on the overall expenditure or time duration or quality. In addition, futuristic approaches like TENS (transcutaneous electrical nerve stimulation) or drug delivery systems can potentially provide non-invasive therapeutic solutions as quick remedies. With the help of AI and other intelligent algorithms, healthcare providers can be more flexible with managing different IoMT devices, leading to enhanced healthcare outcomes, specifically in emergency circumstances [23].

2.8 CHALLENGES IN IOMT

The HIPAA (Healthcare Insurance Portability and Accountability Act) was incorporated by the US government in 1996 to maintain and govern PMI (protected medical information) in addition to adopting authentic digital services. The sustained expansion of IoMT on electronic gadgets generates voluminous data on the networking system, which can also serve as a target for cyberattacks. The increased threat of cybersecurity attacks in the healthcare sector from the use of IoMT-assisted services was first reported in 2015. The outbreak of COVID-19 has also created an ideal opening for the circulation of malware and ransomware. Based on a report, 35% of medical data was hacked in 2019, which increased to 43% in 2021. Data privacy has remained challenging due to the transformed expansion and multifaceted characteristics of IoMT technology. Here, data privacy stands for the transformation, clustering, and backup of records with authenticated access along with the ensuring of security of data [24]. The cybercriminals exploit to hack and gain access to the restricted data. Hence, the challenges to data security include malware attacks, denial-of-service, and ransomware attacks. The edge functionalities of the IoMT framework transmit and receive data on a wireless sensor network (WSN) and exploit a loophole for cyber intrusions. Also, application programs running on a digital platform contain confidentiality violations. Thus, the IoMT system should achieve an additional level of security for the medical data with improved built-in architectures [25]. Thus, there is a prime need for innovative and sophisticated solutions that need to be employed if these devices are indeed utilized universally [26]. The ultimate aim of IoMT systems is to transform the reactionary approach taken by healthcare providers into a proactive and patient-focused approach, which can lead to a positive impact on health and an enhanced quality of medical care [27].

2.9 CONCLUSION

The widespread availability of computational resources and computing power across the globe has paved the way for futuristic or "smart" technological development in various realms of science. The revolution of IoT has profoundly changed the scientific and technological landscape. In this regard, the IoMT is a type of IoT that involves the application of clinical devices and sensors to monitor critical health and physiology-related statistics. Moreover, IoMTs in healthcare settings are increasingly employed for various purposes that affect the quality of our lives [28]. The IoMT platform has massively occupied the healthcare sector and dominated with transformative advancements. The efficiency of IoMT devices lies in accurately predicting possible healthcare outcomes through the monitoring of real-time data of patients. Although the incorporation of IoMT on medical instruments and software-based applications has potentially empowered the healthcare sector, certain limitations and constraints come with IoMT, like security loopholes, data collection and transmission, data confidentiality, and latency issues [29]. The multifaceted characteristics of the IoMT devices pose a significant roadblock in their systemization, exposing security threats. Although the implementation of blockchain mitigates the impact of cyber threats, it improves security and interoperability of IoMT systems. However, the blockchain strategy remained immature and was still limited to the blockchain-based IoMT platforms [30]. With the advancements, the IoMT will make further progress by improving protection, data security, and multimodality processing ability. Hence, the futuristic approach to the IoMT adapts to the current challenges and broadens its range of smart healthcare services.

CONSENT FOR PUBLICATION

None declared.

CONFLICT OF INTEREST

The authors declare no competing financial interest.

ACKNOWLEDGMENT

This chapter was supported by the Department of Biotechnology–National Network Project (DBT-NNP) (Grant No. BT/PR40156/BTIS/137/54/2023); Department of Biotechnology–Bioinformatics Centre (DBT-BIC) (Grant No. (BIC)-No.BT/PR40154/BTIS/137/34/2021) and MoE-STARS (No. MoE-STARS/STARS-2/2023-0966 dt: 29-05-2024).

REFERENCES

1. Gupta, A., and A. Singh. 2023. "Healthcare 4.0: Recent Advancements and Futuristic Research Directions." *Wireless Personal Communications* 129: 933–952. https://doi.org/10.1007/s11277-022-10164-8.
2. Huang, C., J. Wang, S. Wang, and Y. Zhang. 2023. "Internet of Medical Things: A Systematic Review." *Neurocomputing* 557: 126719. https://doi.org/10.1016/j.neucom.2023.126719.
3. Ahmed, S. F., M. S. Sakruque, and N. Ahmed. 2023. "Insights into Internet of Medical Things (IoMT): Data Fusion, Security Issues, and Their Potential Solutions." *Information Fusion* 557: 102060. https://doi.org/10.1016/j.inffus.2023.102060.
4. Hossain, M. S., G. Muhammad, and N. Guizani. 2020. "Explainable AI and Mass Surveillance System-Based Healthcare Framework to Combat COVID-19 Like Pandemics." *IEEE Network* 34 (4): 126–132. https://doi.org/10.1109/MNET.011.2000458.
5. Wagner, A. L. 2019. "The Use and Significance of Vaccination Cards." *Human Vaccines & Immunotherapeutics* 15 (12): 2844–2846. https://doi.org/10.1080/21645515.2019.1625647.
6. El-Saleh, A. A., A. M. Sheikh, M. A. M. Albreem, et al. 2025. "The Internet of Medical Things (IoMT): Opportunities and Challenges." *Wireless Networks* 31: 327–344. https://doi.org/10.1007/s11276-024-03764-8.
7. Ying, H., X. Liu, M. Zhang, et al. 2024. "A Multicenter Clinical AI System Study for Detection and Diagnosis of Focal Liver Lesions." *Nature Communications* 15: 1131. https://doi.org/10.1038/s41467-024-45325-9.

8. Dai, H.-N., H. Wang, G. Xu, J. Wan, M. Imran, and H.-N. Dai. 2019. "Big Data Analytics for Manufacturing Internet of Things: Opportunities, Challenges, and Enabling Technologies." *Enterprise Information Systems* 14: 1–26. https://doi.org/10.1080/17517575.2019.1633689.
9. Razdan, S., and S. Sharma. 2022. "Internet of Medical Things (IoMT): Overview, Emerging Technologies, and Case Studies." *IETE Technical Review* 39 (4): 775–788. https://doi.org/10.1080/02564602.2021.1927863.
10. Gasparin, A. T., C. I. F. Araujo, P. Schmitt, and others. 2022. "Hilab System, a New Point-of-Care Hematology Analyzer Supported by the Internet of Things and Artificial Intelligence." *Scientific Reports* 12: 10409. https://doi.org/10.1038/s41598-022-13913-8.
11. Nasser, N., Q. Emad-Ul-Haq, M. Imran, A. Ali, I. Razzak, and A. Al-Helali. 2023. "A Smart Healthcare Framework for Detection and Monitoring of COVID-19 Using IoT and Cloud Computing." *Neural Computing and Applications* 35 (19): 13775–13789. https://doi.org/10.1007/s00521-021-06396-7.
12. Marzec, M., R. Koprowski, Z. Wróbel, A. Kleszcz, and S. Wilczyński. 2015. "Automatic Method for Detection of Characteristic Areas in Thermal Face Images." *Multimedia Tools and Applications* 74 (12): 4351–4368. https://doi.org/10.1007/s11042-013-1745-9.
13. Khan, A., J. Ali Shah, K. Kadir, W. Albattah, and F. Khan. 2020. "Crowd Monitoring and Localization Using Deep Convolutional Neural Network: A Review." *Applied Sciences* 10 (14): 4781. https://doi.org/10.3390/app10144781.
14. Holland, J., L. Kingston, C. McCarthy, E. Armstrong, P. O'Dwyer, F. Merz, and M. McConnell. 2021. "Service Robots in the Healthcare Sector." *Robotics* 10 (1): 47. https://doi.org/10.3390/robotics10010047.
15. Elkin, D., and V. Vyatkin. 2020. "IoT in Traffic Management: Review of Existing Methods of Road Traffic Regulation." In *Proceedings of the International Conference on Industrial Engineering*, 536–551. Springer. https://doi.org/10.1007/978-3-030-51974-2_50.
16. Kaldoudi, E. 2024. "Smart Hospital: The Future of Healthcare." *Computational and Structural Biotechnology Journal* 24: 87–88. https://doi.org/10.1016/j.csbj.2023.12.011.
17. Kwon, H., S. An, H.-Y. Lee, W. C. Cha, S. Kim, M. Cho, and H.-J. Kong. 2022. "Review of Smart Hospital Services in Real Healthcare Environments." *Healthcare Informatics Research* 28 (1): 3–15. https://doi.org/10.4258/hir.2022.28.1.3.
18. Rahman, M. M., F. Khatun, S. I. Sami, and A. Uzzaman. 2022. "The Evolving Roles and Impacts of 5G-Enabled Technologies in Healthcare: The World Epidemic COVID-19 Issues." *Array* 14: 100178. https://doi.org/10.1016/j.array.2022.100178.
19. Phelan, A. L., R. Katz, and L. O. Gostin. 2020. "The Novel Coronavirus Originating in Wuhan, China: Challenges for Global Health Governance." *JAMA* 323 (8): 709–710. https://doi.org/10.1001/jama.2020.1097.
20. Rahman, M. S., N. C. Peeri, N. Shrestha, R. Zaki, U. Haque, and S. H. Ab Hamid. 2020. "Defending Against the Novel Coronavirus (COVID-19) Outbreak: How Can the Internet of Things (IoT) Help to Save the World?" *Health Policy and Technology* 9 (2): 136–138. https://doi.org/10.1016/j.hlpt.2020.04.005.
21. Nussbaumer-Streit, B., V. Mayr, A. I. Dobrescu, A. Chapman, E. Persad, I. Klerings, G. Wagner, U. Siebert, C. Christof, C. Zachariah, et al. 2020. "Quarantine Alone or in Combination with Other Public Health Measures to Control COVID-19: A Rapid Review." *Cochrane Database of Systematic Reviews* 2020 (4). https://doi.org/10.1002/14651858.CD013574.
22. Adeghe, E., C. Okolo, and O. Ojeyinka. 2024. "A Review of Wearable Technology in Healthcare: Monitoring Patient Health and Enhancing Outcomes." *Open Access Research Journal of Multidisciplinary Studies* 7 (1): 142–148. https://doi.org/10.53022/oarjms.2024.7.1.0019.

23. Jamshidi, M., O. Moztarzadeh, A. Jamshidi, A. Abdelgawad, A. S. El-Baz, and L. Hauer. 2023. "Future of Drug Discovery: The Synergy of Edge Computing, Internet of Medical Things, and Deep Learning." *Future Internet* 15 (4): 142. https://doi.org/10.3390/fi15040142.
24. Dilawar, N., M. Rizwan, F. Ahmad, and S. Akram. 2019. "Blockchain: Securing Internet of Medical Things (IoMT)." *International Journal of Advanced Computer Science and Applications (IJACSA)* 10 (1). https://doi.org/10.14569/IJACSA.2019.0100110.
25. Shafique, K., B. A. Khawaja, F. Sabir, S. Qazi, and M. Mustaqim. 2020. "Internet of Things (IoT) for Next-Generation Smart Systems: A Review of Current Challenges, Future Trends, and Prospects for Emerging 5G-IoT Scenarios." *IEEE Access* 8: 23022–23040. https://doi.org/10.1109/ACCESS.2020.2970118.
26. Bhushan, B., A. Kumar, A. K. Agarwal, A. Kumar, P. Bhattacharya, and A. Kumar. 2023. "Towards a Secure and Sustainable Internet of Medical Things (IoMT): Requirements, Design Challenges, Security Techniques, and Future Trends." *Sustainability* 15 (7): 6177. https://doi.org/10.3390/su15076177.
27. Mathkor, D. Mansor, N. Mathkor, Z. Bassfar, F. Bantun, P. Slama, F. Ahmad, and S. Haque. 2024. "Multirole of the Internet of Medical Things (IoMT) in Biomedical Systems for Managing Smart Healthcare Systems: An Overview of Current and Future Innovative Trends." *Journal of Infection and Public Health* 17 (4): 559–572. https://doi.org/10.1016/j.jiph.2024.01.013.
28. Madakam, S., R. Ramaswamy, and S. Tripathi. 2015. "Internet of Things (IoT): A Literature Review." *Journal of Computer and Communications* 3 (5): 164–173. https://doi.org/10.4236/jcc.2015.35021.
29. Razdan, S., and S. Sharma. 2021. "Internet of Medical Things (IoMT): Overview, Emerging Technologies, and Case Studies." *IETE Technical Review* 39 (4): 775–788. https://doi.org/10.1080/02564602.2021.1927863.
30. Mackey, T. K., T. T. Kuo, B. Gummadi, et al. 2019. "'Fit-for-Purpose?' – Challenges and Opportunities for Applications of Blockchain Technology in the Future of Healthcare." *BMC Medicine* 17: 68. https://doi.org/10.1186/s12916-019-1296-7.

3 Internet of Medical Things

Architecture and Technologies

Gnanasankaran Natarajan,
Sundaravadivazhagan Balasubramanian,
Rakesh Gnanasekaran, and Devika Govindhan

3.1 INTRODUCTION: DETAILED OVERVIEW OF INTERNET OF MEDICAL THINGS (IOMT)

The management, monitoring, and provision of medical services will be completely transformed by the new and more extensive technology that is being applied in healthcare. It is made possible with the advent of the IoMT. IoMT is a collection of healthcare-related electronic gadgets or software, Healthcare systems work together to digitize and expedite medical procedures. This intricate strategy makes use of contemporary technology and the Internet to improve patient care, expedite medical procedures, and enhance general health results. The IoMT, for instance, is a huge collection of intelligent devices connected to the Internet. It gathers, sends, and evaluates health-related data instantly. These gadgets include smart sensors and wearable health monitors, as well as cutting-edge medical equipment that is simple to link online.

The objective is to establish a healthcare system through which physicians can readily obtain critical data, remotely monitor patients, and utilize data to decide on preventive and customized treatment.

3.2 KEY COMPONENTS OF IOMT

- **Medical Devices and Sensors**

IoMT mainly relies on many medical devices equipped with sensors capable of collecting various health data. Examples of these devices include wearable devices, implantable sensors, and tracking devices.

 DOI: 10.1201/9781003476344-3

- **Data Communication**

The foundation of the IoMT is data connectivity; that is made possible via the Internet. Healthcare practitioners can examine health records in real time, thanks to medical gadgets that securely send information to local servers or cloud-based platforms.

- **Data Storage and Processing**

Health data is collected, stored in secure databases, and processed and analyzed using advanced equipment algorithms. Machine learning (ML) and artificial intelligence (AI)-based procedural algorithms play a vital role in getting all relevant insights from large amounts of health information.

- **Interoperability**

Interoperability between various systems and devices is emphasized by IoMT. This promotes a cohesive approach to patient care by guaranteeing ongoing communication and information sharing among all components of the healthcare ecosystem.

- **Security and Privacy**

As the health-related information is sensitive in nature, the IoMT prioritizes maximum security and privileged privacy. Strong encryption, authentication, and provision for control technologies are used to prevent unwanted access to patient information [1].

The IoMT structure is shown in Figure 3.1.

3.3 ASSISTANCE OF IOMT

There are five critical components that support the IoMT. Let us consider them in detail.

3.3.1 Remote Patient Monitoring (RPM)

Medical practitioners can remotely check vital signs and medication, thanks to IoMT's intelligent real-time patient monitoring. RPM is a new era of healthcare within the IoMT that collects and transmits patient data remotely using linked medical devices and technology. As seen in Figure 3.2, this technology allows medical professionals to treat chronic illnesses and compute and track patients' health conditions without making regular in-person visits. RPM makes use of the IoMT's smart device, sensor, and communication technologies to guarantee accurate and continuous patient monitoring on a real-time basis [2].

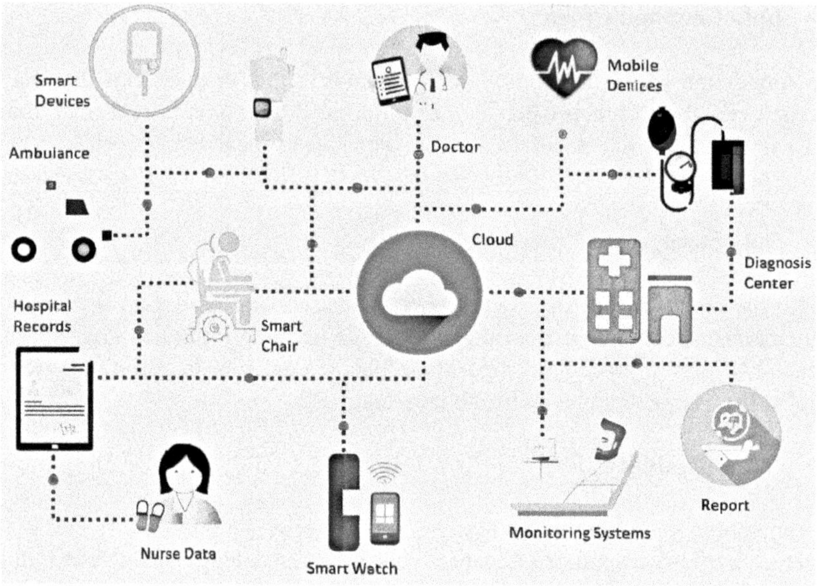

FIGURE 3.1 Structure of IoMT.

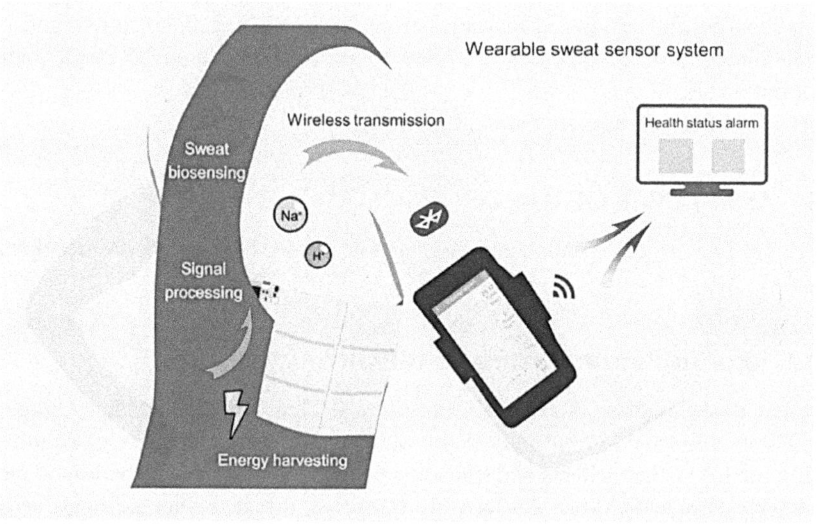

FIGURE 3.2 Smart sensor devices used in healthcare for remote patient monitoring.

3.3.1.1 Key Components of IoMT RPM

- **Wearable Devices and Sensors**

Wearable Health Trackers: Smartwatches, fitness bands, and other wearables outfitted with sensors may track vital indications, including heart rate, activity levels, and sleep patterns.

Medical Sensors: To keep an eye on particular health parameters like blood pressure, oxygen saturation, and glucose levels, special sensors can be integrated into clothing, patches, or implanted devices.

Connectivity

Internet Connectivity: RPM devices are Internet-connected, allowing health data to be transmitted seamlessly to healthcare provider systems.

Wireless Technologies: Bluetooth, Wi-Fi, and other wireless communication technologies allows devices to transmit data securely and in real time.

- **Data Transmission and Storage**
- *Cloud-Based Platforms:* A secured cloud system is where most health data is stored and processed via devices that monitor patients remotely. This ensures that medical professionals may access and analyze the information.
- *Electronic Health Records (EHRs):* Integration with EHR systems allows complete control and continuous maintenance of one's medical history [3].
- **Alerts and Notifications**

Automated Alerts: RPM systems can be set up to alert healthcare practitioners when certain limitations or problem patterns are discovered in patient data. This allows for early action and reduces the risk of problems.

- **Patient Engagement**

Patient Portals: Many RPM systems include a patient portal or mobile application that allows individuals to view their health information. It provides insight into their symptoms and encourages active participation in their care.

Educational Resources: RPM platforms may include educational tools and information to assist patients understand their problems and follow treatment recommendations.

3.3.1.2 Benefits of IoMT RPM

Continuous monitoring enables early detection of changes in health indicators, which allows medical professionals to act quickly to avoid consequences. RPM offers regular monitoring and individualized treatment programs, making it particularly useful for treating long chronic types of conditions such as diabetes, cardiovascular disease, and respiratory disease. By preventing crises and reducing the need for frequent hospital stays, RPM can lower healthcare expenses for both individuals and healthcare systems.

Instead of dealing with repeated clinic visits, patients can control their daily life. This can lead to better patient satisfaction and adherence to the treatment plan. Because RPM collects a wealth of current data, healthcare professionals shall make a causable decision that may lead to more personalized and efficient care. IoMT RPM is a powerful tool in today's healthcare system that encourages proactive and patient action—targeted therapies. The main advantage of IoMT in remote patient observation is that it helps in patent care outcomes for the complete healthcare process [4].

3.3.2 Improved Diagnosis and Treatment

The IoMT refers to the procedure of integrating medical devices to the global web in **order** to collect, share, and analyze health data. Faster and more accurate diagnosis made possible by IoMT data results in treatment programs that are tailored to the individual health profile of each patient. IoMT provides significant support to the healthcare system, leading to more accurate diagnosis and treatment. IoMT helps improve healthcare in the following ways.

- **Remote Monitoring**

IoMT enables remote monitoring of patient health through connected devices. Wearable sensors, smartwatches, and other health monitoring devices can continuously collect important activity levels and other relevant information.

Healthcare providers may remotely monitor patients, identify possible issues early, and take action before they worsen, thanks to this continuous flow of real-time data. Those who are ill will particularly benefit from this.

- **Data Analytics and ML**

IoMT generates vast amounts of health data that may be examined through ML techniques and robust analytics. These technologies are able to identify trends, patterns, and irregularities in data. By using ML techniques, healthcare providers can increase the accuracy of their diagnoses. Disease progression can be predicted with the aid of predictive analytics. Based on the patient's symptoms, treatment can be properly planned and the processes can be optimized.

- **Faster Diagnosis**

IoMT improves the speed and efficiency of diagnosis by improving data transfer between medical devices and healthcare providers. For example, medical imaging systems can send images directly to specialists for rapid review and interpretation. This will help speed up the diagnostic process. It shortens the time taken to start a treatment and ultimately improves patient outcomes.

- **Telemedicine and Telehealth**

The expansion of telemedicine as well as services is significantly influenced by IoMT. Virtual consultations are made possible via connected gadgets. Applications for telemedicine and remote illness monitoring assist medical practitioners in identifying and treating patients irrespective of their physical requirements. It is helpful for patients who live in remote locations, have mobility problems, or are unable to attend in person during emergencies like pandemics.

- **Personalized Medicine**

IoMT facilitates the collection of vast volumes of patient-specific data, enabling medical practitioners to customize treatment plans to meet the needs of each patient. This trend in individualized medicine lowers the likelihood of medication side effects while increasing treatment effectiveness.

- **Better Patient Engagement**

IoMT promotes patient participation in healthcare by giving them access to health information. The patient should be able to get personal health advice and communicate more effectively with their doctors. Greater patient involvement can lead to better compliance in lifestyle changes and overall health outcomes. Integrating IoMT in healthcare can transform the diagnostic and treatment landscape by improving the speed, accuracy, and privacy of treatment which will ultimately lead to better patient care [5].

3.3.3 Enhanced Operational Efficiency

The IoMT boosts operational effectiveness in the healthcare sector by improving communication and maximizing resources through technology. There are several ways that IoMT can improve healthcare efficiency.

> Healthcare workers may remotely observe all medical supplies, assets, and facilities, thanks to IoMT. This may include checking the condition and operation of medical equipment. Inventory level monitoring ensures that critical systems function properly. Remote monitoring reduces the need for physical monitoring. This saves time and cost and enables preventive maintenance to prevent equipment failure.

Medical equipment status can be updated in real time using IoMT devices. This data can be used by predictive maintenance algorithms to forecast failures of equipment or maintenance requirements. This strategy helps healthcare companies plan care more efficiently, reduce downtime, limit disruptions to patient care, and extend the life of medical devices. IoMT improves inventory management by providing up-to-date information on the use and availability of medical supplies and medicines. Automated inspection systems can help prevent overstocks and streamline the supply chain which reduces waste, increases cost-effectiveness, and builds trust in healthcare facilities.

IoMT can improve clinical processes by automating daily procedures and facilitating communication between healthcare providers. For example, patient data produced by IoMT devices can be automatically linked to EHRs, reducing human data entry and the potential for errors. Automating administrative functions, appointment, and billing can improve overall workflow efficiency in healthcare enterprises.

The IoMT encourages the adoption of telehealth services that enable remote treatment by health professionals. This can lead to better utilization of healthcare resources by eliminating the need for a physical office visit.

Telehealth consultation and remote monitoring can help prioritize in-person appointments for patients who need immediate intervention, while routine monitoring and follow-up can be done remotely.

A great deal of health data is produced by the IoMT. By using contemporary analytical methods to examine this data, healthcare organizations can identify trends, learn more about patient demographics, and make well-informed decisions.

Considerable knowledge about operational options, including labor size, property management, and resource allocation, can be gained from the data generated by the IoMT. Whether they are working remotely or in the same institution, IoMT allows healthcare workers to communicate in real time. This enhances care coordination and teamwork.

Effective communication systems can reduce decision-making delays, improve the exchange of important information, and enhance healthcare efficiency by streamlining procedures and resource management and enabling data-driven decision-making. This development will lead to cost-savings, good patient care, and a more curable healthcare system [6].

3.3.4 Proactive Healthcare Management

IoMT that employs technology to track, evaluate, and respond to health data in real time is a key component of predicted individual health management. By preventing and treating illnesses before they worsen, preventive health management enhances general well-being. Here are some examples of how IoMT is supporting predictive healthcare.

IoMT gadgets like networked sensors and wearables provide real-time data to identify anomalies or patterns that can forewarn health issues. Vital signs, including heart rate, blood pressure, and blood sugar levels, are monitored on a daily basis. Healthcare professionals can receive alerts and respond quickly. It allows for proactive management of conditions such as high blood pressure or diabetes. IoMT promotes proactive health management by addressing the importance of medicine. Smart pill dispensers and medication reminders can help people stick to recommended regimens. Good compliance leads to better disease control and reduced risk of outcomes. IoMT's health and well-being apps enable users to measure and manage multiple elements of their well-being, such as exercise, sleep, and nutrition.

These apps provide personalized guidance and actionable information to help people make informed choices about healthy lifestyles.

IoMT enables faster detection of health trends through continuous data collection and analysis. Changes in body type, such as rapid weight changes, sleep disturbance, or increased heart rate can indicate health problems. Early detection can lead to faster healing and slow down the progression of disease and thereby improve health outcomes.

IoMT promotes proactive health management by providing telehealth services. This proactive strategy promotes preventative care and early intervention. It helps reduce the need for reactive healthcare interventions. IoMT can be used to monitor behavioral health indicators of stress and mental well-being. Clothing with biometric sensors can detect physiological signals related to stress. IoMT improves preventive health.

3.3.5 Patient Empowerment

IoMT gadgets like networked sensors and wearables provide real-time data to identify anomalies or patterns that can forewarn of health issues. Vital signs including heart rate, blood pressure, and blood sugar levels are monitored on a daily basis.

Wearable sensors as well as smart health monitors are examples of IoMT devices that allow patients to track their well-being in real time. Health information, activity levels, sleep habits, and other significant health markers all are visible to them. Patients are more conscious of their health state now as they now have access to health information. It enables people to choose their lifestyle with greater knowledge, frequent medication use, and self-care in general. Health professionals and patients can communicate easily, thanks to IoMT. Patients can ask questions, share health information, and get guidance using secure chat platforms and virtual consultations. This open channel of communication fosters a collaborative relationship between patients and healthcare providers. This has led to a rise in patient-centered healthcare and data-driven decision-making.

Medication adherence tools such as smart pill dispensers and medication reminder apps are potential components of the IoMT system. These tools help people stick to their medication plans. IoMT promotes medication adherence. This helps improve disease management and reduce the risk of complications by helping patients participate in their treatment. IoMT helps expand telehealth services by allowing patients to access healthcare remotely. Virtual consultation, remote monitoring, and telemedicine technology are improving access to healthcare, thereby empowering patients, including those who live in remote areas or who have mobility problems, by providing accessible telehealth services.

IoMT helps patients by giving them accessibility to health information in real time, personalized insights, more opportunities to interact with medical professionals, and self-management tools. Better decision-making, greater adherence to treatment plans, and ultimately improved health are the outcomes of this empowerment.

Thus, a new age of combined, patient-focused, and data-based healthcare services is being ushered in by the IoMT, a recent breakthrough in the healthcare industry. As technology advances, IoMT has the potential to significantly influence the next stage of delivery of healthcare and enhance patients' overall well-being worldwide [7].

3.4 IOMT ARCHITECTURE

In order to supply medical data as well as data across the networks, sensors that are medical equipment, and healthcare systems, the IoMT architecture is made up of multiple levels and components. The IoMT design aims to achieve interoperability, security, and efficient information management.

The IoMT architecture's fundamental elements are as follows.

3.4.1 Sensors and Devices

IoMT is based on sensor and healthcare smart devices that give health-related data. These gadgets can be wearables (like smartwatches and fitness trackers), implanted devices, medical sensors, and other networked gadgets that track measurements of vital signs, levels of activity, and other health metrics.

3.4.2 Edge Devices and Gateways

Gateways and edge devices act as a bridge connecting sensors and other devices to the central server or cloud. Before transferring data to the cloud, they locally preprocess and filter it. Edge computing facilitates real-time computation at the device, lowers latency, and conserves bandwidth.

3.4.3 Communication Protocols

There are many communications protocols that facilitate data exchange between any smart system, gateways, and cloud servers. Common IoMT protocols are MQTT, CoAP, and HTTP/HTTPS. These protocols ensure efficient and secure communication [8].

3.4.4 Cloud Infrastructure

The cloud architecture centrally processes, stores, and analyzes the massive volume of data produced by IoMT devices. For healthcare providers along with other stakeholders, cloud-based solutions enable scalability, flexibility, and accessibility. Services like data analytics, ML, and storage options can also be found in cloud settings. The cloud-integrated IoMT architecture is depicted in Figure 3.3.

3.4.5 Security Measures

Healthcare data is sensitive and robust in IoMT architecture. This entails utilizing secure authentication techniques, encrypting data, and adhering to healthcare data

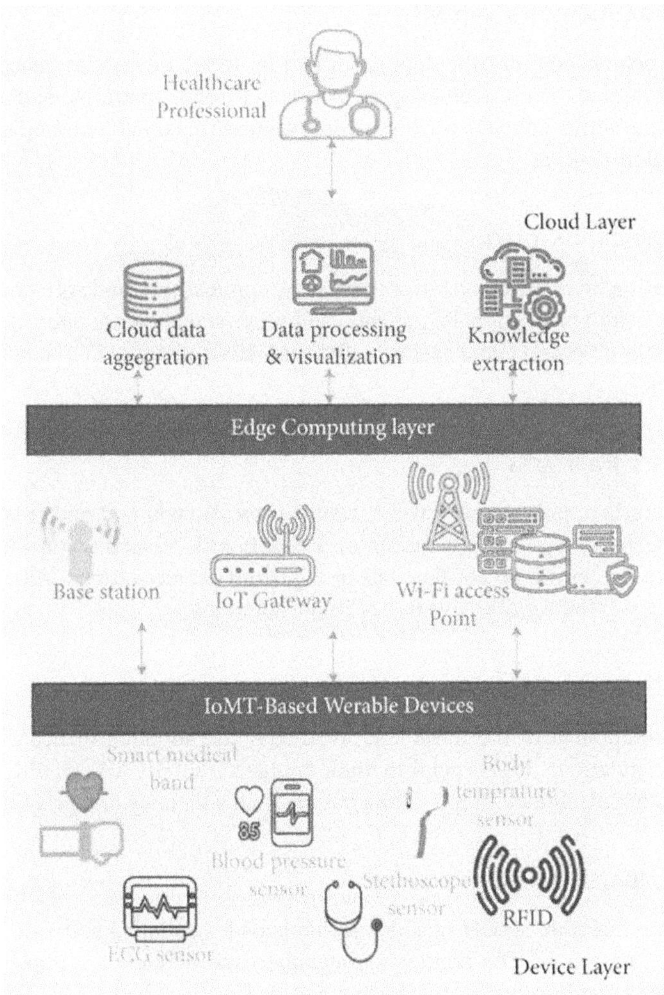

FIGURE 3.3 IoMT architecture integrated with cloud.

protection laws (such as HIPAA in the United States). Patient data availability, confidentiality, and integrity are guaranteed by security mechanisms.

3.4.6 Middleware

Middleware acts as a bridge between different components of the IoMT architecture, which facilitates communication and collaboration. It helps manage data flow, integrate different devices, and ensure compatibility between different technologies.

3.4.7 Data Analytics and ML

These components analyze the data generated by IoMT devices to generate meaningful information. These technologies can detect trends, patterns, and anomalies. It enables predictive analysis for disease prevention, personalized medication, and better decision-making.

3.4.8 Application Layer

The application layer covers the user interfaces, applications, and software solutions with which health professionals, patients, and other stakeholders interact, including mobile apps, web portals, and systems of record. EHR displays and manages health information.

3.4.9 User Interfaces

The user interface provides a way for health professionals and end users to interact with the IoMT system. It consists of a dashboard. Visualization tools and an interface are for setting up notifications or adjusting device settings. An easy-to-use interface is essential for effective use of IoMT solutions.

3.4.10 Regulatory Compliance

A crucial component of the IoMT architecture is the adoption of healthcare standards and regulations. It is crucial to abide by laws like HIPAA, GDPR, and other local requirements. It aids in protecting patient data's security and privacy.

3.4.11 Updates and Maintenance

The IoMT architecture should include mechanisms for updating software, firmware, and security protocols. The regular maintenance and updates are important to fix vulnerabilities and improve system performance.

The IoMT architecture is a tough ecosystem that integrates hardware, software, communication protocols, and security measures to enable efficient collection, transmission, analysis, and use. Health information is a well-designed IoMT architecture that helps improve patient care, streamline healthcare workflows, and improve medical research and care [9].

3.5 IMPORTANCE OF AI IN IOMT

3.5.1 Overview of AI

AI is a process of doing human work without the interference of human intelligence. There are many tasks that AI can do, such as learning, problem-solving, language comprehension, and decision-making. The main objective of AI is to create systems that can imitate, simulate, or reproduce human intelligent functions, allowing them to perform complex tasks independently or with minimal human intervention.

AI systems are designed to study from experience and adapt to changing inputs.

AI is divided into two main types:

- **Narrow /Weak AI**

This kind of process is intended to train a certain population or for a specific objective. It competes in well-defined functions, but its capabilities are limited to those jobs that call for specific programming or training. Virtual personal assistants, image recognition software, and some language translations are a few examples.

- **General/Strong AI**

General AI refers to actual human intelligence. This form of AI is still largely theoretical and has not been achieved.

AI systems employ various techniques and methodologies:

- **Machine Learning**

Actually, ML is a subfield of AI that helps systems perform better on a given task by using statistical models and algorithms.

- **Natural Language Processing (NLP)**

Natural language communication involving computers and humans is made possible by machines' comprehension, production, and recognition of human language.

- **Computer Vision**

The goal of this area of AI is to give machines the ability to understand, analyze, and present information from the outside world, such as pictures and videos.

- **Robotics**

The integration of AI into physical systems that allows machines to do work.

- **Expert Systems**

It is a rule-based process that mimics the prediction-making skills of business. A human expert in a particular field uses a database and inference engine. AI is applied across multiple sectors and domains, including healthcare, finance, education, automotive, and more. It has the potential to evolve the way tasks are performed, automate repetitive processes, and contribute to advancements in technology and society. Nonetheless, as the area develops further, ethical issues, privacy problems, and the need for AI system development and implementation continue to be significant factors [10].

3.5.2 AI with IoMT

AI plays an important role in enhancing the capabilities of IoMT by offering advanced techniques as well as processing capabilities to extract valuable information and thereby improve healthcare operations and patient outcomes.

3.5.2.1 Data Integration and Aggregation

IoMT data collection generates a large volume of health-related data from a variety of sources, including EHRs, medical sensors, and mobile devices. It facilitates the smooth integration and fusion of these disparate data points to produce a comprehensive patient picture.

3.5.2.2 Real-Time Monitoring and Diagnostics

Continuous Monitoring: The algorithms of AI can determine the current data from IoMT devices to observe patient signs, detect abnormally, and provide early signs for potential health conditions.

Diagnostics: Artificial intelligent systems can help in detecting medical conditions by evaluating imaging data (like X-rays and MRIs) and comparing it with historical data and relevant medical literature.

3.5.2.3 Predictive Analytics and Risk Stratification

Risk Assessment: The algorithms of AI can find health risks and stratify patients based on their likelihood of developing certain conditions. This enables proactive and personalized healthcare interventions.

Preventive Measures: AI can identify modern classified patient information. It can recommend preventive measures and lifestyle modifications to reduce the risk of specific health issues.

3.5.2.4 Treatment Personalization

Precision Medicine: AI analyses all types of genetic, clinical, and lifestyle information on treatment plans to each single patient. This ensures that treatments are more effective and have fewer adverse effects.

3.5.2.5 RPM

Telehealth: AI-powered IoMT devices offer sensors for monitoring, allowing doctors to keep an eye on patients' status without making frequent in-person visits.

3.5.2.6 Enhanced Decision Support

Clinical Decision Support Systems (CDSS): AI provides a better healthcare professionals' pattern-making by giving identical data, promotes treatment options, and alerts them to potential issues or contraindications.

3.5.2.7 Efficient Healthcare Operations

Workflow Optimization: AI has the potential to increase overall productivity in healthcare institutions by streamlining administrative duties and closely examining resource distribution.

3.5.2.8 Security and Privacy

Cybersecurity: Given the delicate state of health data, AI is used to improve IoMT network and device security, guard against potential cyber threats, and maintain patient privacy.

3.5.2.9 Research and Development

Drug Discovery: AI helps in the determination of drug identifying processes by discovering large datasets, discovering potential drug persons, and forecasting their effectiveness.

Clinical Trials: By finding qualified candidates, forecasting patient reactions, and enhancing the overall effectiveness of the research process, AI helps improve and expedite clinical trials. By increasing patient outcomes while rendering healthcare more individualized, effective, and accessible, the combination of AI and IoMT holds significant promise for effectively changing the healthcare process. But it also increases challenges in areas like privacy, information protection, and the ethical utilization of AI in healthcare; this requires careful consideration for the technologies to be successfully implemented [11].

3.6 Applications of AI and ML Algorithms within IoMT

To glean insightful information from the vast volumes of health data produced by networked devices, the IoMT heavily relies on AI and ML. This is a comprehensive analysis of how AI and ML are used in IoMT.

AI ALGORITHMS FOR DATA INTEGRATION

- AI methods are used to gather data from a variety of sources, including imaging systems, wearable technology, medical sensors, and EHRs. These methods need managing multiple data formats, regulations, and protocols.
- **Continuous Monitoring with ML Models**

ML models are trained to monitor real-time databases from IoMT devices. These models can recognize common patterns in a patient's vital signs and detect abnormalities that may indicate potential health problems. It allows one to take action early.

- **Image Recognition and Classification**

AI is used in medical imaging to automatically identify and categorize picture patterns. A convolutional neural network (CNN) is frequently employed for tasks like identifying anomalies in X-ray pictures or tumors in radiography imaging.

- **Predictive Modeling**

To forecast the likelihood of disease given a health event or circumstance, ML models have been taught using patient history. This facilitates proactive health intervention and aids in risk categorization.

- **Genomic Analysis with AI**

Genomic data is analyzed by AI to search potential genetic selection that could affect therapy response. The treatment plan can then be improved to be more successful using this information.

- **Pattern Recognition for Remote Monitoring**

Data from RPM can be analyzed by ML algorithms to find trends. It assists medical professionals in monitoring long-term trends in patient health and reacts to departures from the standard.

- **Clinical Decision Support**

AI provides decision support for health professionals by reviewing patient data. It suggests possible diagnosis and recommends treatment options.

- **Workflow Optimization**

AI is used to monitor healthcare workflow by streamlining routine administrative tasks. Scheduling and resource allocation is automated. This helps improve the overall operational efficiency of the healthcare facility.

- **Cybersecurity Measures**

IoMT cybersecurity uses AI algorithms to identify and block potential cyber threats. This includes monitoring network traffic, detecting abnormal behavior, and securing communication channels to protect patient information.

- **Predictive Modeling for Drug Research**

ML is used to analyze biological and chemical data. Accelerate the drug discovery process by predicting potential opportunities and potential drug effectiveness.

- **Selection of Patients for Clinical Trials**

AI helps identify suitable candidates for clinical trials based on certain criteria and optimizes the recruitment process [12].

- **Observations from Textual Data**

Using textual data, the AI discipline of natural language processing (NLP) is utilized to extract helpful data from unstructured EHRs and to gather other data for a more thorough examination and comprehension of the patient's past. The ultimate objective is making healthcare more comprehensive and individualized by using these technologies to enhance patient care and improve health outcomes.

3.7 TYPES OF ML ALGORITHMS APPLIED IN IOMT

ML algorithms serve a significant part in the global IoMT by enabling systems and devices to learn from data, make predictions, and generate meaningful information. IoMT addresses a range of healthcare concerns by utilizing several kinds of ML approaches. The following types of ML algorithms are commonly used in IoMT.

3.7.1 Supervised Learning

A labeled data set, in which the input data is correlated with matching output labels, is the focus of the algorithm in supervised learning. Using labeled medical images from CT, MRI, and X-ray scans, supervised learning is utilized to identify and classify diseases. It is used in predictive modeling for disease development, drug responses, and patient outcomes.

3.7.2 Unsupervised Learning

Unsupervised learning comprises practice models on unlabeled data, and the algorithm identifies similarities and relationships within the information without predefined output labels. Unsupervised learning is used to detect unusual patterns or outliers in health data, signaling potential health issues. This ML algorithm can be applied for grouping patients with similar characteristics or health profiles for personalized treatment plans.

3.7.3 Reinforcement Learning

Reinforcement learning is the study of how the consumers and their environment work together to make decisions. Customers receive feedback in the form of rewards or punishment based on their performance. Reinforcement learning can optimize treatment plans by learning from patient feedback and adjusting interventions over time. The use of reinforcement learning is to adjust monitoring strategies based on patient status and response [13].

3.7.4 Deep Learning

Multilayered neural networks are used in deep learning to automatically recognize features in data. One use of CNNs within the medical image analysis is the detection of anomalies in radiological images. Neural networks (RNNs) and algorithms are used to analyze and extract information from the unstructured text data in EHRs.

3.7.5 Ensemble Learning

Several ML models are used in ensemble learning to improve generalization and overall performance. One of the rare uses of ensemble learning algorithms is to combine similarities from several models to improve the precision and dependability of disease prediction in patient populations.

3.7.6 Online Learning

Online learning involves improving the models continuously as new information becomes available, allowing the system to adapt to changes over time. Online learning is used for updating models in real time as new patient data is collected, ensuring that the system remains current and responsive.

3.7.7 Transfer Learning

Transfer learning leverages subjects to get data from one task to improve performance on multiple but related tasks. It is applied by the knowledge gained from one healthcare domain (e.g., radiology) to improve performance in another (e.g., pathology).

3.7.8 Federated Learning

By evaluating model training on dispersed devices without sharing raw data, cooperative learning protects privacy. In order to keep patient data local and private, blended learning is utilized for training models on data from several healthcare institutions.

The care process, particularly healthcare, input conditions, and intended results are the main topics of the ML process option. Together, these algorithms assess, evaluate, and collect information from health data in IoMT, which eventually contributes to better patient treatment and medical results [14].

3.8 ROLE OF EDGE COMPUTING FOR LOCALIZED DATA PROCESSING

Instead of depending on cloud-based infrastructure, the distributed computing paradigm places computing and data collection closer to the point of data creation. It is especially useful in situations where small spaces, real-time processing, and fast response times are important. Here's how to use edge computing for on-premise data processing to reduce latency and maintain responsiveness to priority.

3.8.1 Proximity to Data Source

Edge computing involves computing resources (servers, processing units, etc.) closer to the location where information is generated. This proximity reduces the physical distance that data must travel, minimizing latency.

3.8.2 Local Data Processing

Although all data is transmitted to a common cloud server for processing, edge computing enables processing to take place on edge devices or edge servers. This would be especially advantageous for time-sensitive applications that require immediate processing.

3.8.3 Real-Time Analytic

Real-time analysis of the data generated by edge devices is possible. This is crucial for applications where real-time data insights can lead to quick decisions and actions, such as autonomous vehicles, medical treatment, and industrial IoT (Internet of Things).

3.8.4 Reduced Bandwidth Usage

The data produced by edge devices can be analyzed in real time. This is essential for applications like industrial IoT (Internet of Things), medical care, and driverless cars wherein real-time data insights can result in prompt choices and actions [15].

3.8.5 Event-Triggered Responses

Edge computing enables event-based response. Certain actions are performed immediately when a specific event occurs. This is especially important in applications such as smart cities, where edge devices can respond in real time to events such as traffic expressions, security events, or changes in the environment.

3.8.6 Autonomous Systems

Drones and self-driving cars are examples of personal systems that depend heavily on edge computing. In order to navigate and react to the environment while depending on distant cloud resources, these system functions must be able to make snap judgments according to local sensor inputs.

3.8.7 Offline Operation

Edge devices can continue to function even if they lose connection to the central cloud. In cases where continuous connection cannot be guaranteed, this is important to ensure that critical functions can still function on the machine.

3.8.8 Privacy and Security

Edge computing addresses security and privacy concerns by keeping data remotely on the device. For applications like healthcare, it is especially important to communicate with multiple points of contact rather than just one. When managing sensitive patient data, the utmost confidentiality must be upheld.

3.8.9 Scalability

Horizontal scaling is made possible by edge processing. If more data processing is required, more edge devices might be added as needed. This enables the system to scale flexibly in response to demand [16].

3.9 IMPACT OF BLOCKCHAIN TECHNOLOGY IN MAINTAINING THE SECURED DATA OF HEALTHCARE

Blockchain technology's unique features—such as encryption techniques, decentralization, transparency, and immutability—have led to its application in the healthcare sector to enhance the privacy and confidentiality of medical data. Here are some ways that blockchain improves the privacy and security of health data.

3.9.1 Decentralization

A healthcare manager oversees a centralized database that houses patient data in the conventional healthcare system. Because of their centralization, malicious actors find these databases to be a desirable target. Each member has a copy of the complete blockchain, which is operated by a decentralized network of nodes. Single points of failures are less complicated as a result of this decentralization. This makes it harder for unauthorized parties to compromise the system as a whole.

3.9.2 Immutability

After being input or modified, data can be deleted or altered from centralized databases, which could lead to issues like unauthorized changes or data breaches. A blockchain's data is immutable, meaning once a block has been included to the chain, it cannot be altered or tampered with. This ensures that health data is accurate and resistant to unauthorized modifications.

3.9.3 Data Ownership and Control

Patients often do not have control over their health information, and obtaining it can require complex procedures and intermediaries. Blockchain allows patients to better manage their health information. Patients can authorize certain parties to access their information and track who accessed it and when. It puts patient data ownership and privacy at the center [17].

3.9.4 Smart Contracts for Consent Management

Managing patients' consent to share data can be difficult and imprecise. Smart contracts are self-executing contracts whose terms are written in code. In healthcare, smart contracts can be used to manage patient requests.

3.9.5 Encryption and Cryptographic Techniques

Data is usually encrypted in transit, but can also be stored in plain text in a database. Blockchain platforms use encryption technology to protect data. Each network participant has a private key and data is encrypted and decrypted using this key. Add a layer of security to your health data, whether it is in transit or at rest.

3.9.6 Transparent Auditing

Monitoring access to health data in centralized systems is difficult and unclear. Blockchain provides a clear record and traceability of all transactions. Every input, change, or addition to government data is recorded in a block, providing a transparent and transparent audit trail. This function builds accountability and trust in the system.

3.9.7 Interoperability

Health data is often separated in different health systems, creating connectivity issues. Blockchain promotes collaboration by providing a standardized, secure, and scalable way for multiple institutions, including hospitals, clinics, and research institutes, to share health data.

3.9.8 Private and Permissioned Blockchains

Public blockchains are secure, but may not be suitable for all healthcare situations due to privacy concerns. Private and permissioned blockchains limit authorized participants, ensuring that only trust entities with clear permission can access the network. In the healthcare sector, wherein data privacy is crucial, this is particularly crucial.

By combining these characteristics, blockchain technology offers a potent solution for handling sensitive data in the healthcare sector and resolves a number of privacy and security concerns pertaining to healthcare data framework for health security [18].

3.10 CONCLUSION AND FUTURE SCOPE

An innovative advancement in healthcare, the IoMT focuses on state-of-the-art technologies to improve patient care, automate medical processes, and deliver optimal treatment. Today, gathering, analyzing, and making decisions regarding data is made simpler by the architecture of IoMT, which is characterized by connected medical systems and devices.

The potential use of IoMT for healthcare purposes is growing in importance as a result of ongoing advancements and discoveries. Predictive analytics, individualized treatment regimens, and effective healthcare operations are made possible by the combination of AI and ML. By lowering latency, edge computing enables targeted data processing and quick reactions to important events. Blockchain ensures the security and integrity of health data, giving patients more control over their data.

As the IoMT ecosystem grows, more flexibility, standardization, and interoperability may become possible. This technological convergence has a chance to revolutionize healthcare practices, advance a patient-centered approach, and create opportunities for innovative solutions to address the constantly growing issues facing the medical industry. The probable future of IoMT in healthcare is defined by a commitment to better medical results, data security, and the continuous pursuit of innovations that enhance people's overall well-being and the effectiveness of healthcare systems [19].

REFERENCES

1. Razdan, S., & Sharma, S. (2022). Internet of medical things (IoMT): Overview, emerging technologies, and case studies. *IETE Technical Review*, 39(4), 775–788.
2. Ghubaish, A., Salman, T., Zolanvari, M., Unal, D., Al-Ali, A., & Jain, R. (2020). Recent advances in the Internet-of-Medical-Things (IoMT) systems security. *IEEE Internet of Things Journal*, 8(11), 8707–8718.
3. Hu, F., Xie, D., & Shen, S. (2013, August). On the application of the internet of things in the field of medical and health care. In *2013 IEEE international conference on green computing and communications and IEEE Internet of Things and IEEE cyber, physical and social computing* (pp. 2053–2058). IEEE.

4. Ajagbe, S. A., Awotunde, J. B., Adesina, A. O., Achimugu, P., & Kumar, T. A. (2022). Internet of medical things (IoMT): Applications, challenges, and prospects in a data-driven technology. In *Intelligent healthcare: Infrastructure, algorithms and management* (pp. 299–319). Springer.
5. Gatouillat, A., Badr, Y., Massot, B., & Sejdić, E. (2018). Internet of medical things: A review of recent contributions dealing with cyber-physical systems in medicine. *IEEE Internet of Things Journal*, 5(5), 3810–3822.
6. Joyia, G. J., Liaqat, R. M., Farooq, A., & Rehman, S. (2017). Internet of medical things (IoMT): Applications, benefits and future challenges in healthcare domain. *Journal of Communications*, 12(4), 240–247.
7. Thamilarasu, G., Odesile, A., & Hoang, A. (2020). An intrusion detection system for internet of medical things. *IEEE Access*, 8, 181560–181576.
8. Wei, K., Zhang, L., Guo, Y., & Jiang, X. (2020). Health monitoring based on internet of medical things: Architecture, enabling technologies, and applications. *IEEE Access*, 8, 27468–27478.
9. Sun, L., Jiang, X., Ren, H., & Guo, Y. (2020). Edge-cloud computing and artificial intelligence in internet of medical things: Architecture, technology and application. *IEEE Access*, 8, 101079–101092.
10. Manickam, P., Mariappan, S. A., Murugesan, S. M., Hansda, S., Kaushik, A., Shinde, R., & Thipperudraswamy, S. P. (2022). Artificial intelligence (AI) and internet of medical things (IoMT) assisted biomedical systems for intelligent healthcare. *Biosensors*, 12(8), 562.
11. Chakraborty, C., Banerjee, A., Garg, L., & Rodrigues, J. J. (2020). Internet of medical things for smart healthcare. In *Studies in big data* (Vol. 80). Cham, Switzerland: Springer.
12. Oniani, S., Marques, G., Barnovi, S., Pires, I. M., & Bhoi, A. K. (2021). Artificial intelligence for internet of things and enhanced medical systems. In *Bio-inspired neurocomputing* (pp. 43–59). Springer.
13. Aminizadeh, S., Heidari, A., Toumaj, S., Darbandi, M., Navimipour, N. J., Rezaei, M., ... Unal, M. (2023). The applications of machine learning techniques in medical data processing based on distributed computing and the Internet of Things. *Computer Methods and Programs in Biomedicine*, 241, 107745.
14. Rodriguez-Rodriguez, I., Rodriguez, J. V., Shirvanizadeh, N., Ortiz, A., & Pardo-Quiles, D. J. (2021). Applications of artificial intelligence, machine learning, big data and the internet of things to the COVID-19 pandemic: A scientometric review using text mining. *International Journal of Environmental Research and Public Health*, 18(16), 8578.
15. Yu, W., Liang, F., He, X., Hatcher, W. G., Lu, C., Lin, J., & Yang, X. (2017). A survey on the edge computing for the Internet of Things. *IEEE Access*, 6, 6900–6919.
16. Ai, Y., Peng, M., & Zhang, K. (2018). Edge computing technologies for Internet of Things: A primer. *Digital Communications and Networks*, 4(2), 77–86.
17. Zubaydi, H. D., Chong, Y. W., Ko, K., Hanshi, S. M., & Karuppayah, S. (2019). A review on the role of blockchain technology in the healthcare domain. *Electronics*, 8(6), 679.
18. Chenthara, S., Ahmed, K., Wang, H., Whittaker, F., & Chen, Z. (2020). Healthchain: A novel framework on privacy preservation of electronic health records using blockchain technology. *PLoS One*, 15(12), e0243043.
19. Bhushan, B., Kumar, A., Agarwal, A. K., Kumar, A., Bhattacharya, P., & Kumar, A. (2023). Towards a secure and sustainable Internet of Medical Things (IoMT): Requirements, design challenges, security techniques, and future trends. *Sustainability*, 15(7), 6177.

4 Tapestry of Promise and Peril

NLP, AI, and IoMT in Healthcare Transformation – A Review

Baranidharan S., Sujatha Ravinatayana Bhat, Sonal Devesh, and Gayathry S. Warrier

4.1 INTRODUCTION

Healthcare is at a crossroads. On one hand, AI, NLP, and IoMT hold much promise for personalized care, remote monitoring, and data-driven insights. Shadows of security, privacy, and ethical concerns loom large. This chapter delves into the tapestry these technologies weave, examining their potential to revolutionize patient care while acknowledging the hurdles that threaten to unravel it. Explore the threads of NLP, AI, and IoMT, unraveling challenges and weaving a future of healthcare that is not only technologically advanced but also ethical, inclusive, and empowering for all. As healthcare stands at a crossroads, a confluence of technologies emerges, promising to revolutionize patient care. Natural language processing (NLP), artificial intelligence (AI), and the Internet of Medical Things (IoMT) compose a future full of promise—Kumar and Gond (2023) imagine NLP breaking the communication barriers between humans and machines through chatbots and virtual assistants, while Manickam et al. (2022) demonstrated AI-centric systems that improve treatment plans through IoMT inputs. In one breath, Sato et al. (2022) have painted a decentralized clinical trials scenario with wide patient participation into drug development, thanks to IoMT. However, there is hope and darkness along with it. Ajagbe et al. (2022) raise fears regarding the susceptibility of IoMT toward security breaches and privacy violations, and Rawat (2022) calls out to security through blockchain integrity. Decentralized trials only remain in an ambiguous ethical landscape, as explained by Shakeel et al. (2023), while needing more oversight to protect the safety of patients and maintain ethical behavior. These technologies, in review, discuss how they can shape patient care through these advancements while recognizing which obstacles might unravel it. With insights from Dwivedi et al. (2022) on optimizing resource allocation through IoMT, Razdan and

DOI: 10.1201/9781003476344-4

Sharma (2022) on real-time data collection, and Wal et al. (2022) advocating for IoMT as the future of healthcare, we discuss practical and research implications, opening the door to a future where these technologies empower, not exploit.

4.2 BRIDGING THE GAP BETWEEN THE PROMISE AND PERILS OF NLP, AI, AND IOMT IN HEALTHCARE

These factors include limited access to healthcare, inefficient use of data, and outdated methods in clinical trials, which prevent proper healthcare delivery. NLP, AI, and IoMT are, however, beacons of hope, promising a future of personalized care, remote monitoring, and data-driven insights. However, security, privacy, and regulatory hurdles remain. A multipronged approach is needed: (1) Develop secure, privacy-preserving NLP and AI algorithms for IoMT data analysis. (2) Implement strong IoMT infrastructure with blockchain-based security and interoperability standards. (3) Foster regulatory frameworks for decentralized clinical trials based on IoMT data while ensuring patient safety and ethical conduct. In this way, we can overcome these challenges and unlock the true potential of NLP, AI, and IoMT for a future of accessible, personalized, and data-driven healthcare.

4.3 AI AND IOMT IN SMART HEALTHCARE

Sharma (2023) explored the possibility of a personalized telemedicine approach using artificial intelligence (AI), robotics, and the Internet of Medical Things (IoMT) in smart healthcare. In this study, the author indicated that this system could provide some benefits, including better access of patients to healthcare services, advanced monitoring and diagnostic capabilities, and tailored treatment regimens. However, one of the main challenges is those of data privacy and security along with regulatory obstacles. Ramakrishnan et al. (2023) presented a roadmap for AI and IoMT in smart healthcare: current applications and future perspectives. The authors discuss those areas where AI and IoMT have the potential to bring about a qualitative impact on patients, such as remote patient monitoring, chronic disease management, and precision medicine. The authors underlined the need for collaboration among researchers, clinicians, and policymakers to ensure the ethical and responsible development of these technologies. Kalinaki et al. (2024) reviewed the cybersecurity challenges associated with the use of AI and IoMT in smart cities, focusing on smart healthcare applications. The identified vulnerabilities included data breaches, device hijacking, and malware attacks. The authors further recommended the adoption of robust security measures, which include secure communication protocols, data encryption, and access control mechanisms, to minimize these risks.

Rufai et al. (2024) studied cyberattacks on AI-enabled IoMT systems in smart healthcare. They reported that these systems were being targeted by attackers because the data they collect and store are sensitive. The authors recommended that a defense-in-depth approach that combines technical, physical, and administrative safeguards should be adopted. Saravanan and Prabha (2024) present a comprehensive study on the deployment of edge computing and AI systems in smart healthcare during the

COVID-19 era. They determined that these technologies were critical support systems for the remote monitoring of patients, tracing contacts, and distributing vaccines. The authors have concluded that, although edge computing and AI will transform healthcare delivery, more investments and developments will be needed. Jolly et al. (2023) looked into the potential of AI-enabled IoMT in medical applications. They discussed some use cases such as real-time patient monitoring, early disease detection, and personalized interventions. They emphasized the necessity of interoperability and standardization of IoMT devices and data formats to seamlessly integrate AI-powered solutions into clinical workflows. These articles present valuable insights regarding the potential and challenges of applying AI and IoMT in smart healthcare. It is indicated that these technologies hold the potential for transforming healthcare delivery through personalized, remote, and data-driven care.

4.4 AI AND IOMT: APPLICATIONS, CHALLENGES, AND FUTURE TRENDS

Jamshidi et al. (2023) envisioned a future where edge computing, IoMT, and deep learning converge to transform drug discovery. They envisioned AI analyzing real-time patient data from IoMT devices to personalize drug targets and optimize clinical trials. Shah and Khang (2023) focused on the role of IoMT in the transformation of digital healthcare. They mentioned its potential for improving patient monitoring, chronic disease management, and remote consultations, thus making care more accessible and efficient. Sinha et al. (2023) discussed the big data analytics and IoMT combination with explainable AI in the healthcare sector. They supported explainable AI models to be applied in order to increase the reliance and transparency associated with AI-driven healthcare decisions. Kumar et al. (2023) presented a scalable architecture for the Indian smart healthcare system using IoMT. The scalable architecture would have ensured secure patient data management with secure transactions among healthcare providers. Osama et al. (2023) presented an overview of IoMT in Healthcare 4.0, including trends, requirements, challenges, and future research directions. They seem to state that for the successful implementation of IoMT, standardization, interoperability, and strong security protocols are in order.

Idrees et al. (2023) discussed the applications of deep learning in IoMT networks for the fight against the COVID-19 pandemic. They mentioned some possible applications such as virus spread prediction, contact tracing, and personalized patient care. Monteiro et al. (2023) provided a general overview of IoMT applications, including the potential to enhance disease diagnosis, treatment planning, and medication adherence. They also mentioned challenges such as data privacy, cybersecurity, and user acceptance. Natarajan et al. (2023) proposed a new framework for improving security and energy efficiency in IoMT for Healthcare 5.0. The framework intended to optimize resource allocation, avoid cyberattacks, and prolong device battery life. Muheidat and Tawalbeh (2023) analyzed AIoMT (AI and IoMT) applications, challenges, and future trends. They identified areas such as real-time monitoring, personalized medicine, and remote surgery as promising avenues for AIoMT adoption, while highlighting concerns about data privacy, ethical considerations, and potential job displacement. Mohan et al. (2023) proposed a revolutionary framework to secure and privatize genomic data in 5G healthcare using blockchain-based IoMT. This framework aimed to ensure data integrity, patient control, and auditable access logs. Majeed et al. (2023) reviewed IoMT applications in smart healthcare in terms of the ISA (Intelligent Secure Architecture) framework. They elaborated on how ISA enables the secure exchange of data, interoperability, and collaboration between IoMT devices and healthcare systems. These articles give an optimistic view about the prospect of IoMT in changing the healthcare map in the future. It can make medicine more personalized, accessible, and easy for everyone to get proper care. However, the following challenges must be addressed to enable successful implementation of IoMT, such as cybersecurity, data privacy, and ethical considerations. The more research goes on and those concerns are reduced, the ability of IoMT to usher in a new patient-centric, data-driven, intelligent healthcare era grows.

Sharma et al. (2023) proposed the use of deep graph neural networks as a method for the detection of replication attacks in IoMT, where an attacker can attack data integrity. Their results demonstrated that the model was highly precise in identifying the mentioned attacks. Yazid (2023) discussed the various cybersecurity and privacy issues pertaining to IoMT, including data breaches, unauthorized access, and vulnerabilities on devices. They stressed the requirement for strong security controls to safeguard confidential patient information and maintain confidentiality. Kiran et al. (2023) presented a detailed review of security and privacy issues in IoMT. They addressed possible threats, risk assessment techniques, and different security controls to counter such risks. Yang (2024) explored privacy issues related to ML-based fall prediction models in geriatric care under IoMT. They pointed to the surveillance potential and data abuse possibilities, further recommending ethical recommendations and privacy-sensitive approaches. Anitha et al. 2023 provided an AI security model for defense of IoMT devices and network from cyberattack. Figure. 4.1 -The developed model utilizes the AI techniques on intrusion detection, anomaly detection, and live threat mitigation in real time. Khan et al. (2023) designed an IoMT system for remote monitoring of patients. The system visually presents patient data streams, so healthcare providers can easily understand the status of the patient's health and take necessary decisions. Jayachitra et al. (2023) discussed how AI is an enabler of smart healthcare solutions within IoMT. They described the predictive analytics, medical image analysis, and real-time decision support AI may bring to better the outcomes for patients. These articles emphasize that security and privacy are crucial to IoMT. There are a number of techniques that are being researched for the above reasons, including AI-driven models, deep learning, and visualization tools. Ensuring robust security and protecting patient privacy remain critical issues for the future development of IoMT in healthcare.

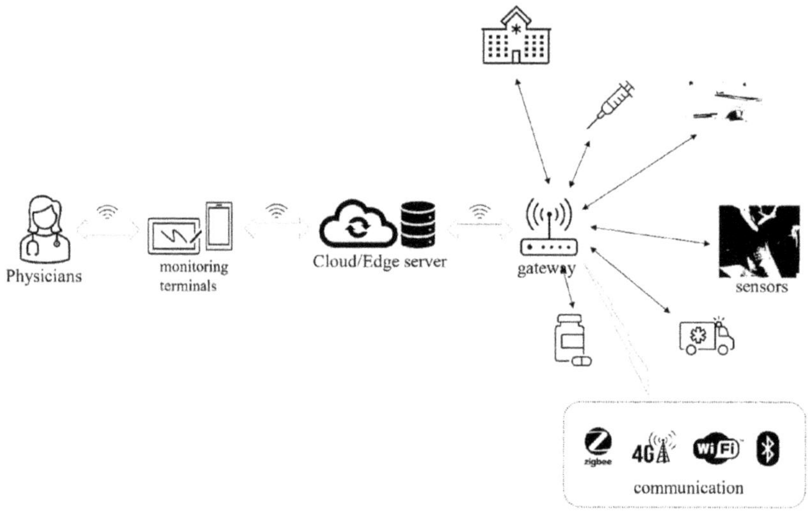

FIGURE 4.1 A simple prototype of an IoMT system.

4.5 CYBER-BIOSECURITY AND BLOCKCHAIN TECHNOLOGY IN IOMT

Pandey, Maurya, and Chiong's Data Modelling and Analytics for the Internet of Medical Things (2023) explored the intersection of healthcare and advanced data analytics, emphasizing how IoMT devices generate actionable insights for patient care. The volume exhibited challenges in big data handling, security, and interoperability while presenting frameworks for efficient data modeling. By integrating AI, machine learning, and predictive analytics, it demonstrates how connected medical systems could improve diagnostics, treatment, and personalized care. Overall, the book positions IoMT as a transformative force in building intelligent, data-driven healthcare ecosystems. Taherdoost (2023) investigates the potential use of blockchain in IoMT as it enhances the security, transparency, and traceability of healthcare applications. Envisaged blockchain-based platforms could enable secure sharing of patient information, automated claims processing, and improved medication management. Rao et al. (2023) proposed a low-cost and dependable IoMT topology for minimizing the cost of maintenance and deployment. Their proposed approach took into account density in device, network coverage, and energy consumption to optimize network infrastructure for real-world healthcare scenarios. Elgabry (2023) recommended a "cyber-biosecurity by design" approach to the development of IoMT. The approach focused on the integration of security measures at the design stage itself, accounting for both cyber threats and biological risks from medical devices and their data. Singh et al. (2023) suggested an Industry 4.0–enabled IoMT solution for secure and cost-effective smart patient care. The "medicine pouch," consisting of sensors and AI capacity, is intended for real-time health monitoring, medication adherence, and the delivery of personalized treatment. Sakly et al. (2022) discussed blockchains technologies in the use of IoMT-based healthcare systems, especially in the COVID-19 pandemic. They argued that blockchain could be able to provide for secure and transparent data sharing, contact tracing, and support vaccination efforts.

Badri et al. (2023) and Garg et al. (2023) demonstrated the BIoMT architecture: a blockchain-based framework to increase information security within IoMT systems. BIoMT focused on privacy of collected data, non-accessibility issues, and authenticity of medical information collected from devices using IoMT. Garg et al. (2023) designed a secure communication model for IoMT systems using an AI approach. This solution applied ML-based algorithms to identify anomalies in data communication, thus protecting the patient data from cyberattacks. Parihar et al. (2023) explored the adaptation of IoMT with point-of-care biosensing devices for infectious disease diagnosis. This, they believed, would better prepare pandemics since, due to quick diagnosis with the tracking of the disease in real-time and personalized intervention of treatment, it would be much easier. Ameen et al. (2023) presented a detailed review of the prospects and challenges related to AI, blockchain, and cybersecurity in IoMT. The authors emphasized that these technologies need to be utilized holistically in order to tap into the complete potential of IoMT while addressing security concerns and promoting ethical AI development. Such articles paint a very promising picture regarding how blockchain, security, and AI synergistically transform IoMT into a robust and secure platform for the future of healthcare. Addressing the data privacy issues, providing the best of robust security, and responsibly incorporating AI will allow IoMT to transform healthcare delivery for the delivery of personalized, data-driven, and accessible care to all.

4.6 IOMT ON E-HEALTHCARE PERFORMANCE

Huang et al. in 2023 performed an all-encompassing review of IoMT, which included its architecture, applications, challenges, and future directions. They outlined IoMT as a great transformer in healthcare delivery through the remote monitoring, personalized medicine, and effective disease management among others. Patra et al. in 2022 adopted a cloud-integrated architecture of IoMT for smart healthcare systems. They highlighted the cloud's capacity to process large amounts of data from IoMT devices, which would allow for data storage, analysis, and real-time insights for clinicians. Khatib et al. (2023) examined the effects of IoMT on e-healthcare performance and discussed how blockchain can improve smart contracts. They believed that blockchain's immutability and transparency could create trust and accountability in healthcare transactions. Alkatheiri and Alghamdi (2023) discussed how blockchain can strengthen IoMT cybersecurity. They introduced blockchain-based, secured data sharing, and access control framework for protection against IoMT network-based cyberattacks to patient privacy. Banday and Bhat (2022) highlighted the idea of healthcare as an inclusive endeavor and addressed IoMT toward neglecting diseases with the development of IoMT-based solutions such as remote diagnosis and monitoring as well as drug delivery in deprived zones. Kamalov et al. (2023) mentioned challenges and solutions with respect to IoMT privacy and security. They came out with the major requirements which were needed for building a secure and trusted IoMT ecosystem: user consent, data anonymization, and intrusion detection.

Mathur et al. (2022) discussed a range of healthcare applications of machine learning in the context of IoMT. These include predictive analytics, disease risk

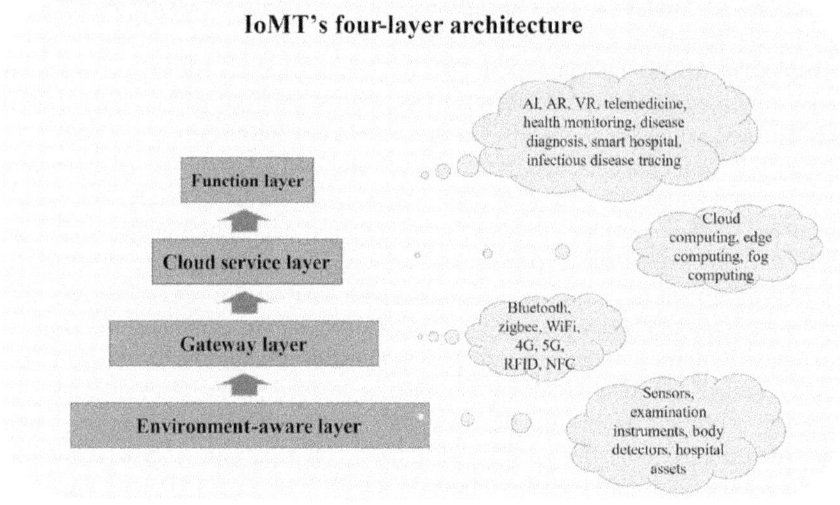

FIGURE 4.2 IoMT's four-layer architecture.

assessment, and personal treatment plans that could potentially change the game for patient care. Ejiyi et al. (2023) also offered a thorough review of IoMT's place in healthcare management. They explored its potentials in resource optimization, remote consultation, and the real-time patient data analysis in improving the healthcare delivery efficiencies. Shrotriya et al. (2023) discussed the applicability of IoMT in the healthcare domain in conjunction with a big data processing framework called Apache Spark. He demonstrated how a huge amount of IoMT could be analyzed in Spark, to enable researchers glean insights for prevention of diseases, personalized medicine, and better patient care. Azim et al. (2022) explained the other applications of IoT in healthcare rather than IoMT. These authors further extended it to e-Health services, assisted living facilities, and e-Wellness initiatives to promote preventive care and patient empowerment. According to Awotunde et al. (2023), IoMT can enhance smart healthcare systems. They presented ideas to facilitate monitoring health real-time, remote surgery assistance, and personalized interventions by IoMT for better patient outcomes. Si-Ahmed et al. (2023) focused their research on intrusion detection methods by machine learning over IoMT networks. They summarized several algorithms and techniques for detection and mitigation of cyberattacks on IoMT in order to achieve data security with patient safety. These articles thus paint a good picture of what IoMT promises to transform about healthcare. They emphasize how IoMT IoMT's four-layer architecture, with the support of cloud computing, blockchain, machine learning, and robust security measures can transform healthcare delivery, making it more accessible, personalized, and data-driven (Figure 4.2). With ongoing research and development, IoMT promises to empower patients, improve healthcare efficiency, and ultimately lead to a healthier future for all. Patra et al. (2022) emphasized secure data sharing, remote monitoring, and scalable health services, while also noting challenges around privacy and interoperability. It offered practical insights into building efficient, technology-driven healthcare systems.

4.7 LEDGER TECHNOLOGY (BLOCKCHAIN) IN e-HEALTHCARE

Bhattacharya et al. (2023) added that federated learning is a privacy-preserving method to train machine learning models on IoMT data. Federated learning could be helpful for collaborative analysis of medical data, respecting patient privacy, toward optimal disease prediction and personalized care. Gupta et al. (2023) presented BIDS (blockchain and intrusion detection system coalition) as a method to secure IoMT networks. BIDS incorporated blockchain's immutability and transparency to implement secure data storage and intrusion detection to ensure overall improved resilience of the IoMT network. Moujahid et al. (2023) systematically surveyed the development of smart healthcare through IoMT and edge–cloud computing. It cited the interoperability between the technologies that allow for real-time processing, low latency, and efficient utilization of resources in efficient healthcare systems delivery. Chaudhury and Sau (2023) proposed a blockchain-enabled IoMT system for breast cancer detection. Their system used blockchain for the secure storage of mammogram images and distributed diagnostic results to authorized healthcare providers, thus ensuring faster diagnosis and collaborative care. Dhanda et al. (2023) discussed 6G technology as a prospect for IoMT. They visualized 6G's ultra-reliable and high-bandwidth capabilities as empowering remote surgery, real-time health monitoring, and seamless integration of medical devices into the healthcare delivery system.

Deshmukh et al. (2022) described the applications of distributed ledger technology, also known as blockchain in e-Healthcare. They said that blockchain could ensure data integrity, enhance traceability, and automate insurance claims processing, creating trust and transparency in healthcare transactions. Zhou et al. (2022) proposed a new rate splitting technique for time minimization in IoMT health monitoring systems. This approach has tried to increase data transmission speed by ensuring that data quality would improve faster, enabling efficient collection and analysis of health data. Sahapudeen et al. (2023) has developed a complete review of 10 deep learning approaches for IoMT. Herein, several applications have been explained such as anomaly detection, disease prediction, and personalized medicine and shown deep learning potential as the unlocking device to unlock meaningful IoMT-based information. In conclusion, these articles paint a very promising picture for the future of IoMT in healthcare. They show how, empowered by federated learning, blockchain, and advanced AI techniques, IoMT can address security concerns, optimize data utilization, and personalize healthcare experiences. With research advancing and these technologies converging, IoMT is set to unlock a data-driven, secure, and patient-centric future for healthcare.

4.8 NATURAL LANGUAGE PROCESSING IN HEALTHCARE

Kumar and Gond (2023) highlighted that NLP may revolutionize the healthcare sector. They talked about the applications of NLP such as medical chatbots, virtual assistants, and automated report analysis that will provide better patient–clinician communication, personalized care plans, and efficient drug discovery. Shakeel et al. (2023) carried out an extensive survey on the effect of COVID-19 on the healthcare sector. They analyzed global market implementations, telemedicine adoption, and the security and privacy concerns. Their conclusion pointed out that the post-pandemic period would require an enhanced healthcare infrastructure and data protection policies. Dwivedi et al. (2022) carried out a systematic review of IoMT applications in building smart healthcare systems. They identified the areas of remote patient monitoring, chronic disease management, and precision medicine where IoMT could be used to optimize resource allocation, personalize treatment plans, and enhance healthcare outcomes. Razdan and Sharma (2022) provided an overview of IoMT, covering its architecture, emerging technologies, such as wearables and implantable, and real-world case studies. The authors concluded that IoMT holds the promise of revolutionizing the delivery of healthcare by allowing for real-time data collection, remote diagnostics, and personalized interventions. These articles are a vivid illustration of how technology is shaping the future of healthcare. They also highlight the potential of NLP in automating tasks, making communication easier, and extracting useful insights from medical data. In addition, the COVID-19 pandemic has pointed out the necessity of agile and resilient healthcare systems, where IoMT can contribute to remote monitoring, data-driven decision-making, and personalized care delivery. These technologies have vast potential to make healthcare more accessible, efficient, and, at the end, better for patients as research and development continue.

4.9 AI AND IOMT IN INTELLIGENT HEALTHCARE

Manickam et al. (2022) suggested AI- and IoMT-powered biomedical systems toward intelligent healthcare. They felt that the upcoming AI algorithms would analyze data collected by IoMT devices to provide real-time patient monitoring and predictive diagnostics along with the personalization of treatment. This would help improve clinical decision-making and patient outcomes. Sato et al. (2022) discussed the use of IoMT in DCTs. They presented ideas on how to enable direct, peer-to-peer collection and exchange of patient information by IoMT devices to improve remote engagement at lower costs, while preserving information confidentiality. Regulatory frameworks would then be needed in order to properly address ethical as well as logistical issues for DCTs. Ajagbe et al. (2022) systematically reviewed IoMT applications, challenges, and potential. They identified areas like remote patient monitoring, chronic disease management, and personalized medicine where IoMT would actually make a big change in healthcare delivery. At the same time, they emphasized that the issues of security, privacy, and interoperability have to be addressed to achieve successful IoMT implementation. Rawat (2022) reviewed blockchain technology used in e-supply chains for IoMT devices. They argued that immutability and transparency in blockchain would ensure the secure sharing of data, tracing of device origin, and combating counterfeits, thereby furthering patient safety and trust in IoMT-based healthcare systems. Lahby et al. (2023) explored how Artificial Intelligence and the Internet of Health Things can strengthen pandemic response through predictive modeling, real-time monitoring, and resource optimization. The book balances technical insights with ethical and social considerations, making it a useful reference for sustainable digital health strategies.

Wal et al. (2022) urged IoMT to be the future of healthcare. They discussed the potential of IoMT in removing geographical barriers, empowering patients, and optimizing the allocation of resources, thus ensuring a more accessible, efficient, and patient-centric healthcare ecosystem. Kim et al. (2022) developed a case study on the implementation of IoMT in hospital communication. They illustrated how the devices of IoMT could facilitate real-time communication among medical staff, track the inventory of medical equipment, and monitor patient vitals to improve the efficiency of the workflow and coordination of care in the hospital setting. The articles show great promise in depicting the coming together of AI, IoMT, and decentralized clinical trials to reshape healthcare. It gives hope to how these technologies could make personalized medicine, optimize clinical processes, and democratize access to health. Though the challenges persist regarding data security, privacy, and regulatory frameworks, the collective efforts of researchers, healthcare providers, and policymakers can pave the way for a future where IoMT and AI empower a healthier world.

4.10 METHODOLOGY

The systematic search was performed using relevant keywords in major academic databases such as PubMed, Scopus, and Google Scholar from 2022 to 2024. Search terms used were as follows: "natural language processing," "artificial intelligence," "Internet of Medical Things," "healthcare," "challenges," and "opportunities." Inclusion Criteria

Articles were selected according to the following criteria such as Concerned to the topics of NLP, AI, and IoMT in healthcare, Original research or comprehensive review articles, Published in peer-reviewed journals within the last five years, Conducted in English, Qualitative Synthesis: all articles are carefully read and main points and conclusions summarized. Summary data is tabled in matrices to facilitate thematic synthesis.

4.11 DISCUSSION

The article "A Future Woven with NLP, AI, and IoMT: Promises and Perils in Healthcare Transformation" provides a compelling picture of the future of healthcare with NLP, AI, and IoMT converging to change the face of patient care. NLP holds the promise of unlocking the hidden secrets in medical jargon and enabling chatbots and virtual assistants to bridge the communication gap while personalizing care plans. AI, powered by IoMT data, sees a future of real-time patient monitoring, predictive diagnostics, and precision medicine, where treatments are tailored to individual needs. Decentralized clinical trials, enabled by IoMT, promise faster drug development and wider patient participation. But amidst this optimism, shadows lurk. Security and privacy concerns loom large as IoMT devices collect sensitive data. Can this data remain safe from breaches and misuse? Decentralized trials' regulatory frameworks are still in their infancy, and this places ethical conduct and patient safety in a gray area. The specter of inequality looms large: Will these technologies make the already present disparities worse, pushing underprivileged communities further into the periphery?

Bridging this gap between possibility and peril requires a multipronged approach. First, security and privacy must be woven into the very fabric of NLP and AI algorithms. Secure enclaves, federated learning, and robust anonymization techniques can protect sensitive data while enabling valuable insights. Second, IoMT infrastructure needs an overhaul. Blockchain's immutable ledger can ensure data integrity and provenance, fostering trust and transparency. Interoperability standards need to be created so that devices and systems can communicate freely, thus eliminating data silos. Lastly, the regulatory landscape needs a revolution of clear guidelines for decentralized trials which include patient safety and ethical considerations without stifling the innovator. Collaboration between researchers, policymakers, and healthcare providers should ensure regulations empower rather than stifle.

At the end of it all, it is all about inclusiveness. Bridge the digital divide and allow everyone to enjoy these technologies. Educational initiatives and community engagement would empower patients and healthcare workers. The road ahead is paved with challenges, but the potential rewards are immense. By responsibly harnessing the power of NLP, AI, and IoMT, they weave a future in which healthcare is not only accessible but also personalized, data-driven, and empowering for all. Let us accept this challenge with cautious optimism because the health and well-being of generations depend on it.

4.12 PRACTICAL IMPLICATIONS

- Create user-friendly NLP interfaces: Develop chatbots and virtual assistants that are accessible to patients with varying technical skills and literacy levels. Use clear, concise language while avoiding medical jargon.
- Introduce AI-triage systems: Introduce AI algorithms in analyzing patient data that prioritize urgent cases, optimize resource allocation, and reduce wait times.
- Decentralized pilot clinical trials: Initiate small-scale trials with strong ethics control and data protection guarantees to collect real-world evidence, refining the protocol.
- Investment in IoMT Infrastructure.
- Infrastructure for healthcare settings: upgrades for secure networks, interoperable devices, and data storage solutions that are privacy-compliant.
- Train healthcare professionals in AI and IoMT: To enable them to correctly interpret the outputs of AI, analyze IoMT data, and use these technological interventions for better patient care.
- Engage in patient education and awareness: Educate patients on their rights over their data, enable patients to participate in research using IoMT, and involve them actively in AI-enabled healthcare.

4.13 IMPLICATIONS OF RESEARCH

- Investigate privacy-preserving NLP: Algorithm development toward extracting insights from medical data where patients' anonymity is preserved and unauthorized access is prevented.
- Research-explainable AI applications in healthcare: Develop AI models with transparent reasoning that explains how a model makes its decisions,

which creates more trust among and acceptance by patients and health professionals.

- Ethical considerations in decentralized clinical trials: In relation to data ownership, right to information, and the potential possibility of exploitation of the vulnerable.
- Assess the cost-effectiveness of IoMT interventions: Analyze the financial impact of implementing IoMT technologies on healthcare systems and patient outcomes.
- Investigate the social and psychological impact of AI and IoMT: Explore how these technologies affect patient–clinician relationships, healthcare worker well-being, and broader societal dynamics.
- Develop interoperable standards for IoMT devices: Bridge the gap between manufacturers and healthcare providers by establishing common protocols for data exchange and device communication.

4.14 CONCLUSION

The tapestry of the future of healthcare is being woven with NLP, AI, and IoMT threads. This chapter, along with the wider study from which it is drawn, reveals the lay of the land—both enormous potential and pressing problems ahead. These articles paint vivid pictures about unlocking medical jargon with NLP, personalized care with AI, and real-time monitoring and decentralized clinical trials with IoMT. These promise a future where healthcare is accessible, data-driven, and personalized. However, shadows lurk amidst this optimism. Security, privacy, ethical considerations, and regulatory hurdles threaten to unravel this delicate tapestry. Bridging this gap requires a multipronged approach: secure, privacy-preserving NLP, and AI algorithms are the foundation for responsible data analysis. Robust IoMT infrastructure with blockchain-based security and interoperability standards is the warp of this future. Clear and ethical frameworks for decentralized trials form the weft; therefore, safety and trust will get woven into every fiber. The success of this transformation is based on inclusion, so bridging the digital divide and empowering both patients and healthcare workers can give life to the far-reaching words of NLP, AI, and IoMT: not being the tools of the privileged few but threads strengthening the weave of healthcare for all. The road ahead will be challenging, but the potential rewards are immense. By embracing cautious optimism and collaborative action, we can weave a future where healthcare is not just accessible but is also personalized, data-driven, and empowering for all. Let us not shy away from this responsibility, as the health and well-being of generations yet to come depends on the very threads we choose to weave today.

REFERENCES

Ajagbe, Sunday Adeola, Joseph Bamidele Awotunde, Ademola Olusola Adesina, Philip Achimugu, and T. Ananth Kumar. 'Internet of Medical Things (IoMT): Applications, Challenges, and Prospects in a Data-Driven Technology'. In *Intelligent Healthcare*, 299–319. Singapore: Springer Nature Singapore, 2022. https://doi.org/10.1007/978-981-16-8150-9_14.

Alkatheiri, Mohammed Saeed, and Ahmed S. Alghamdi. 'Blockchain-Assisted Cybersecurity for the Internet of Medical Things in the Healthcare Industry'. *Electronics* 12, no. 8 (11 April 2023): 1801. https://doi.org/10.3390/electronics12081801.

Ameen, Aya Hamid, Mazin Abed Mohammed, and Ahmed Noori Rashid. 'Dimensions of Artificial Intelligence Techniques, Blockchain, and Cyber Security in the Internet of Medical Things: Opportunities, Challenges, and Future Directions'. *Journal of Intelligent Systems* 32, no. 1 (10 April 2023). https://doi.org/10.1515/jisys-2022-0267.

Anitha, C., C. R. Komala, C. V. Vivekanand, S. D. Lalitha, and S. Boopathi. 'Artificial Intelligence Driven Security Model for Internet of Medical Things (IoMT)'. In *2023 3rd International Conference on Innovative Practices in Technology and Management (ICIPTM)*, 1–7. IEEE, 2023.

Awotunde, Joseph Bamdele, Chinmay Chakraborty, Muyideen AbdulRaheem, Rasheed Gbenga Jimoh, Idowu Dauda Oladipo, and Akash Kumar Bhoi. 'Internet of Medical Things for Enhanced Smart Healthcare Systems'. In *Implementation of Smart Healthcare Systems Using AI, IoT, and Blockchain*, 1–28. Elsevier, 2023. https://doi.org/10.1016/b978-0-323-91916-6.00009-6.

Azim, Mohammad Abdul, Ethel Merry, Jigmey Gyalmo, and Zulfikar Alom. 'IoT in E-Health, Assisted Living, and E-Wellness'. In *The Internet of Medical Things (IoMT) and Telemedicine Frameworks and Applications*, 17–38. IGI Global, 2022. https://doi.org/10.4018/978-1-6684-3533-5.ch002.

Badri, Sahar, Sana Ullah Jan, Daniyal Alghazzawi, Sahar Aldhaheri, and Nikolaos Pitropakis. 'BIoMT: A Blockchain-Enabled Healthcare Architecture for Information Security in the Internet of Medical Things'. *Computer Systems Science and Engineering* 46, no. 3 (2023): 3667–84. https://doi.org/10.32604/csse.2023.037531.

Banday, Mohammad Tariq, and Lubna Bhat. 'Towards Building Internet-of-Things-Inclusive Healthcare for Neglected Tropical Diseases'. In *Advances in Medical Technologies and Clinical Practice*, 39–75. IGI Global, 2022. https://doi.org/10.4018/978-1-6684-3533-5.ch003.

Bhattacharya, P., A. Verma, and S. Tanwar. *Federated Learning for Internet of Medical Things*. Edited by Pronaya Bhattacharya, Ashwin Verma, and Sudeep Tanwar. London, England: CRC Press, 2023. https://books.google.at/books?id=sTW9EAAAQBAJ.

Chaudhury, Sushovan, and Kartik Sau. 'A Blockchain-Enabled Internet of Medical Things System for Breast Cancer Detection in Healthcare'. *Healthcare Analytics* 4, no. 100221 (December 2023): 100221. https://doi.org/10.1016/j.health.2023.100221.

Deshmukh, Atharva, Amit Kumar Tyagi, Harshadi Hansora, and Sanjana Chelat Menon. 'Applications of Distributed Ledger (Blockchain) Technology in E-Healthcare'. In *The Internet of Medical Things (IoMT) and Telemedicine Frameworks and Applications*, 248–61. IGI Global, 2022. https://doi.org/10.4018/978-1-6684-3533-5.ch013.

Dhanda, Sumit Singh, Tarun Kumar Sharma, Brahmjit Singh, Poonam Jindal, and Deepak Panwar. '6G-Enabled Internet of Medical Things'. In *Lecture Notes in Networks and Systems*, 75–84. Lecture Notes in Networks and Systems. Singapore: Springer Nature Singapore, 2023. https://doi.org/10.1007/978-981-19-9858-4_7.

Dwivedi, Ruby, Divya Mehrotra, and Shaleen Chandra. 'Potential of Internet of Medical Things (IoMT) Applications in Building a Smart Healthcare System: A Systematic Review'. *Journal of Oral Biology and Craniofacial Research* 12, no. 2 (March 2022): 302–18. https://doi.org/10.1016/j.jobcr.2021.11.010.

Ejiyi, Chukwuebuka, Zhen Qin, Makuachukwu Bennedith Ejiyi, Grace Ugochi Nneji, Happy Nkanta Monday, Favour Amarachi Agu, Thomas Ugochukwu Ejiyi, Chidinma Diokpo, and Chiduzie Obed Orakwue. 'The Internet of Medical Things in Healthcare Management: A Review'. *Journal of Digital Health* (28 June 2023): 30–62. https://doi.org/10.55976/jdh.22023116330-62.

Elgabry, Mariam. 'Towards Cyber-Biosecurity by Design: An Experimental Approach to Internet-of-Medical-Things Design and Development'. *Crime Science* 12, no. 1 (17 February 2023). https://doi.org/10.1186/s40163-023-00181-8.

El Khatib, Mounir, Haitham M. Alzoubi, Samer Hamidi, Muhammad Alshurideh, Ali Baydoun, and Ahmed Al-Nakeeb. 'Impact of Using the Internet of Medical Things on E-Healthcare Performance: Blockchain Assist in Improving Smart Contract'. *ClinicoEconomics and Outcomes Research: CEOR* 15 (1 June 2023): 397–411. https://doi.org/10.2147/CEOR.S407778.

Garg, Neha, Rajat Petwal, Mohammad Wazid, D. P. Singh, Ashok Kumar Das, and Joel J. P. C. Rodrigues. 'On the Design of an AI-Driven Secure Communication Scheme for Internet of Medical Things Environment'. *Digital Communications and Networks* 9, no. 5 (October 2023): 1080–89. https://doi.org/10.1016/j.dcan.2022.04.009.

Gupta, K., K. D. Gupta, D. Kumar, G. Srivastava, and D. K. Sharma. 'BIDS: Blockchain and Intrusion Detection System Coalition for Securing Internet of Medical Things Networks'. *IEEE Journal of Biomedical and Health Informatics*, 2023: 1–9. https://doi.org/10.1109/JBHI.2023.3325964.

Huang, Chenxi, Jian Wang, Shuihua Wang, and Yudong Zhang. 'Internet of Medical Things: A Systematic Review'. *Neurocomputing* 557, no. 126719 (November 2023): 126719. https://doi.org/10.1016/j.neucom.2023.126719.

Idrees, Ahsan K., Baraa T. Hasan, and Saba K. Idrees. 'Deep Learning for Combating COVID-19 Pandemic in Internet of Medical Things (IoMT) Networks: A Comprehensive Review'. *Advanced AI and Internet of Health Things for Combating Pandemics*, 57, 2023.

Jamshidi, Mohammad (behdad), Omid Moztarzadeh, Alireza Jamshidi, Ahmed Abdelgawad, Ayman S. El-Baz, and Lukas Hauer. 'Future of Drug Discovery: The Synergy of Edge Computing, Internet of Medical Things, and Deep Learning'. *Future Internet* 15, no. 4 (7 April 2023): 142. https://doi.org/10.3390/fi15040142.

Jayachitra, S., A. Prasanth, S. Hariprasath, R. Benazir Begam, and M. Madiajagan. 'AI Enabled Internet of Medical Things in Smart Healthcare'. In *Engineering Cyber-Physical Systems and Critical Infrastructures*, 141–61. Cham: Springer International Publishing, 2023. https://doi.org/10.1007/978-3-031-31952-5_7.

Jolly, Lochan, Niket Amoda, and K. Mishra. 'Artificial Intelligence-Enabled IOMT for Medical Application'. In *Handbook of Research on Artificial Intelligence and Soft Computing Techniques in Personalized Healthcare Services*, 3–32. New York: Apple Academic Press, 2023. https://doi.org/10.1201/9781003371250-2.

Kalinaki, K., M. Fahadi, A. A. Alli, W. Shafik, M. Yasin, and N. Mutwalibi. 'Artificial Intelligence of Internet of Medical Things (AIoMT) in Smart Cities: A Review of Cybersecurity for Smart Healthcare'. In *Handbook of Security and Privacy of AI-Enabled Healthcare Systems and Internet of Medical Things*, 271–92, 2024.

Kamalov, Firuz, Behrouz Pourghebleh, Mehdi Gheisari, Yang Liu, and Sherif Moussa. 'Internet of Medical Things Privacy and Security: Challenges, Solutions, and Future Trends from a New Perspective'. *Sustainability* 15, no. 4 (10 February 2023): 3317. https://doi.org/10.3390/su15043317.

Khan, Mudassar Ali, Ikram Ud Din, Byung-Seo Kim, and Ahmad Almogren. 'Visualization of Remote Patient Monitoring System Based on Internet of Medical Things'. *Sustainability* 15, no. 10 (16 May 2023): 8120. https://doi.org/10.3390/su15108120.

Kim, Boseul, Sunghae Kim, Min Lee, Hyukjae Chang, Eunjeong Park, and Taehwa Han. 'Application of an Internet of Medical Things (IoMT) to Communications in a Hospital Environment'. *Applied Sciences (Basel, Switzerland)* 12, no. 23 (25 November 2022): 12042. https://doi.org/10.3390/app122312042.

Kiran, Ravi, Ashish Kumbhare, Piyush Kumar Thakur, and Shashank Mane. 'Security and Privacy in the Internet of Medical Things (IoMT)'. In *Advances in Healthcare Information Systems and Administration*, 1–27. IGI Global, 2023. https://doi.org/10.4018/978-1-6684-5422-0.ch001.

Kumar, Adarsh, and Anjali Gond. 'Natural Language Processing: Healthcare Achieving Benefits via Nlp'. *ScienceOpen*, 2 August 2023. https://doi.org/10.14293/pr2199.000280.v1.

Kumar, Ravinder, Ritu Rana, and Sunil Kumar Jha. 'Scalable Blockchain Architecture of Internet of Medical Things (IoMT) for Indian Smart Healthcare System'. In *Engineering Cyber-Physical Systems and Critical Infrastructures*, 231–59. Cham: Springer International Publishing, 2023. https://doi.org/10.1007/978-3-031-31952-5_11.

Lahby, Mohamed, Virginia Pilloni, Jyoti Sekhar Banerjee, and Mufti Mahmud. *Advanced AI and Internet of Health Things for Combating Pandemics*. Cham, Switzerland: Springer Nature, 2023. https://books.google.at/books?id=jxbNEAAAQBAJ.

Majeed, F., M. Nazir, and J. Schneider. 'ISA: Internet of Medical Things (IoMT) in Smart Healthcare and Its Applications: A Review'. In *2023 3rd International Conference on Artificial Intelligence (ICAI)*, 129–35. IEEE, 2023.

Manickam, Pandiaraj, Siva Ananth Mariappan, Sindhu Monica Murugesan, Shekhar Hansda, Ajeet Kaushik, Ravikumar Shinde, and S. P. Thipperudraswamy. 'Artificial Intelligence (AI) and Internet of Medical Things (IoMT) Assisted Biomedical Systems for Intelligent Healthcare'. *Biosensors* 12, no. 8 (25 July 2022): 562. https://doi.org/10.3390/bios12080562.

Mathur, Garima, Anjana Pandey, and Sachin Goyal. 'Applications of Machine Learning in Healthcare'. In *The Internet of Medical Things (IoMT) and Telemedicine Frameworks and Applications*, 177–95. IGI Global, 2022. https://doi.org/10.4018/978-1-6684-3533-5.ch009.

Monteiro, Ana Carolina Borges, Reinaldo Padilha França, Rangel Arthur, and Yuzo Iano. 'An Overview of the Internet of Medical Things (IoMT): Applications, Benefits, and Challenges'. In *Security and Privacy Issues in Internet of Medical Things*, 83–98. Elsevier, 2023. https://doi.org/10.1016/b978-0-323-89872-0.00009-5.

Moujahid, Fatima Ezzahra, Siham Aouad, and Mostapha Zbakh. 'Smart Healthcare Development Based on IoMT and Edge-Cloud Computing: A Systematic Survey'. In *Lecture Notes on Data Engineering and Communications Technologies*, 575–93. Cham: Springer Nature Switzerland, 2023. https://doi.org/10.1007/978-3-031-27762-7_52.

Muheidat, Fadi, and Loai A. Tawalbeh. 'AIoMT Artificial Intelligence (AI) and Internet of Medical Things (IoMT)'. In *Computational Intelligence for Medical Internet of Things (MIoT) Applications*, 33–54. Elsevier, 2023. https://doi.org/10.1016/b978-0-323-99421-7.00013-1.

Natarajan, Rajesh, Gururaj Harinahallo Lokesh, Francesco Flammini, Anitha Premkumar, Vinoth Kumar Venkatesan, and Shashi Kant Gupta. 'A Novel Framework on Security and Energy Enhancement Based on Internet of Medical Things for Healthcare 5.0'. *Infrastructures* 8, no. 2 (2 February 2023): 22. https://doi.org/10.3390/infrastructures8020022.

Osama, Manar, Abdelhamied A. Ateya, Mohammed S. Sayed, Mohamed Hammad, Paweł Pławiak, Ahmed A. Abd El-Latif, and Rania A. Elsayed. 'Internet of Medical Things and Healthcare 4.0: Trends, Requirements, Challenges, and Research Directions'. *Sensors (Basel, Switzerland)* 23, no. 17 (25 August 2023): 7435. https://doi.org/10.3390/s23177435.

Pandey, R., P. Maurya, and R. Chiong. *Data Modelling and Analytics for the Internet of Medical Things*. Edited by Rajiv Pandey, Pratibha Maurya, and Raymond Chiong. London, England: Taylor & Francis, 2023. https://books.google.at/books?id=CQPmEAAAQBAJ.

Parihar, Arpana, Shalu Yadav, Mohd Abubakar Sadique, Pushpesh Ranjan, Neeraj Kumar, Ayushi Singhal, Vedika Khare, Raju Khan, Sathish Natarajan, and Avanish K. Srivastava. 'Internet-of-Medical-Things Integrated Point-of-Care Biosensing Devices for Infectious Diseases: Toward Better Preparedness for Futuristic Pandemics'. *Bioengineering & Translational Medicine* 8, no. 3 (May 2023): e10481. https://doi.org/10.1002/btm2.10481.

Patra, Manoj Kumar, Anisha Kumari, Bibhudatta Sahoo, and Ashok Kumar Turuk. 'Smart Healthcare System Using Cloud-Integrated Internet of Medical Things'. In *Exploring the Convergence of Computer and Medical Science Through Cloud Healthcare*, 60–83. IGI Global, 2022. https://doi.org/10.4018/978-1-6684-5260-8.ch004.

Ramakrishnan, Swamynathan, S. Jijitha, and T. Amudha. 'Roadmap of AI and IoMT in Smart Healthcare: Current Applications and Future Perspectives'. In *Internet of Medical Things in Smart Healthcare*, 137–61. New York: Apple Academic Press, 2023. https://doi.org/10.1201/9781003369035-8.

Rao, C. M., G. Prasuna, H. K. Chapala, N. Jeebaratnam, D. Navulla, and A. Verma. 'Designing a Reliable and Cost-Effective Internet of Medical Things (IoMT) Topology to Minimize the Maintenance and Deployment Cost'. In *2023 Fifth International Conference on Electrical, Computer and Communication Technologies (ICECCT)*, 1–07. IEEE, 2023.

Rawat, Romil. 'A Systematic Review of Blockchain Technology Use in E-Supply Chain in Internet of Medical Things (IoMT)'. *International Journal of Computations, Information and Manufacturing (IJCIM)* 2, no. 2 (21 November 2022). https://doi.org/10.54489/ijcim.v2i2.119.

Razdan, Sahshanu, and Sachin Sharma. 'Internet of Medical Things (IoMT): Overview, Emerging Technologies, and Case Studies'. *IETE Technical Review* 39, no. 4 (4 July 2022): 775–88. https://doi.org/10.1080/02564602.2021.1927863.

Rufai, A. U., E. P. Fasina, C. O. Uwadia, A. T. Rufai, and A. L. Imoize. 'Cyberattacks against Artificial Intelligence-Enabled Internet of Medical Things'. In *Handbook of Security and Privacy of AI-Enabled Healthcare Systems and Internet of Medical Things*, 191–216. CRC Press, 2024.

Sahapudeen, Fathima Fathima, T. Vigneswari, and S. K. Mohan. 'Deep Learning Approaches for IoMT.' In *Data Modelling and Analytics for the Internet of Medical Things*, 153–170. CRC Press, 2023.

Sakly, Houneida, Mourad Said, Ahmed A. Al-Sayed, Chawki Loussaief, Rachid Sakly, and Jayne Seekins. 'Blockchain Technologies for Internet of Medical Things (BIoMT) Based Healthcare Systems: A New Paradigm for COVID-19 Pandemic'. In *Trends of Artificial Intelligence and Big Data for E-Health*, 139–65. Cham: Springer International Publishing, 2022. https://doi.org/10.1007/978-3-031-11199-0_8.

Saravanan, K., and G. L. Prabha. 'Edge Computing and Artificial Intelligence Systems Adopted in Smart Healthcare: A Comprehensive Survey in Real-Time COVID-19 Pandemic'. In *Internet of Medical Things in Smart Healthcare*, 99–118. Apple Academic Press, 2024.

Sato, Takahiro, Hikaru Ishimaru, Takuya Takata, Hajime Sasaki, and Mayumi Shikano. 'Application of Internet of Medical/Health Things to Decentralized Clinical Trials: Development Status and Regulatory Considerations'. *Frontiers in Medicine* 9 (6 June 2022): 903188. https://doi.org/10.3389/fmed.2022.903188.

Shah, Vrushank, and Alex Khang. 'Internet of Medical Things (IoMT) Driving the Digital Transformation of the Healthcare Sector'. In *Data-Centric AI Solutions and Emerging Technologies in the Healthcare Ecosystem*, 15–26. Boca Raton: CRC Press, 2023. https://doi.org/10.1201/9781003356189-2.

Shakeel, Tanzeela, Shaista Habib, Wadii Boulila, Anis Koubaa, Abdul Rehman Javed, Muhammad Rizwan, Thippa Reddy Gadekallu, and Mahmood Sufiyan. 'A Survey on COVID-19 Impact in the Healthcare Domain: Worldwide Market Implementation,

Applications, Security and Privacy Issues, Challenges and Future Prospects'. *Complex & Intelligent Systems* 9, no. 1 (2023): 1027–58. https://doi.org/10.1007/s40747-022-00767-w.

Sharma, Amit, Pradeep Kumar Singh, Alexey Tselykh, and Alexander Bozhenyuk. 'Internet of Medical Things (IoMT) Application for Detection of Replication Attacks Using Deep Graph Neural Network'. In *Lecture Notes in Electrical Engineering*, 267–82. Lecture Notes in Electrical Engineering. Singapore: Springer Nature Singapore, 2023. https://doi.org/10.1007/978-981-19-9876-8_21.

Sharma, Kiran. 'Personalized Telemedicine Utilizing Artificial Intelligence, Robotics, and Internet of Medical Things (IoMT)'. In *Handbook of Research on Artificial Intelligence and Soft Computing Techniques in Personalized Healthcare Services*, 301–23. New York: Apple Academic Press, 2023. https://doi.org/10.1201/9781003371250-17.

Shrotriya, L., K. Sharma, D. Parashar, K. Mishra, S. S. Rawat, and H. Pagare. 'Apache Spark in Healthcare: Advancing Data-Driven Innovations and Better Patient Care'. *International Journal of Advanced Computer Science and Applications* 14, no. 6 (2023): 608–16.

Shyam Mohan, J. S., Guddeti Theekshana, and Guddeti Likhit Kumar Reddy. 'Revolutionalizing Internet of Medical Things for Blockchain-based 5G Healthcare Security and Privacy for Genomic Data'. In *Privacy Preservation of Genomic and Medical Data*. Wiley, 17 October 2023. https://doi.org/10.1002/9781394213726.ch8.

Si-Ahmed, Ayoub, Mohammed Ali Al-Garadi, and Narhimene Boustia. 'Survey of Machine Learning Based Intrusion Detection Methods for Internet of Medical Things'. *Applied Soft Computing* 140, no. 110227 (June 2023): 110227. https://doi.org/10.1016/j.asoc.2023.110227.

Singh, Sourav, Sachin Sharma, Shuchi Bhadula, and Seshadri Mohan. 'Industry 4.0 Internet of Medical Things Enabled Cost Effective Secure Smart Patient Care Medicine Pouch'. In *New Horizons for Industry 4.0 in Modern Business*, 149–70. Cham: Springer International Publishing, 2023. https://doi.org/10.1007/978-3-031-20443-2_7.

Sinha, Anurag, Den Whilrex Garcia, Biresh Kumar, and Pallab Banerjee. 'Application of Big Data Analytics and Internet of Medical Things (IoMT) in Healthcare with View of Explainable Artificial Intelligence: A Survey'. In *Internet of Things*, 129–63. Cham: Springer International Publishing, 2023. https://doi.org/10.1007/978-3-031-08637-3_8.

Taherdoost, Hamed. 'Blockchain-Based Internet of Medical Things'. *Applied Sciences (Basel, Switzerland)* 13, no. 3 (18 January 2023): 1287. https://doi.org/10.3390/app13031287.

Wal, Pranay, Ankita Wal, Neha Verma, Rohini Karunakakaran, and Anupriya Kapoor. 'Internet of Medical Things – the Future of Healthcare'. *The Open Public Health Journal* 15, no. 1 (30 December 2022). https://doi.org/10.2174/18749445-v15-e221215-2022-142.

Yang, Russell. 'Privacy and Surveillance Concerns in Machine Learning Fall Prediction Models: Implications for Geriatric Care and the Internet of Medical Things'. *AI & Society* 39, no. 4 (August 2024): 1969–73. https://doi.org/10.1007/s00146-023-01655-8.

Yazid, Ahmed. 'Cybersecurity and Privacy Issues in the Internet of Medical Things (IoMT)'. *Eigenpub Review of Science and Technology* 7, no. 1 (3 April 2023): 1–21. https://studies.eigenpub.com/index.php/erst/article/view/3.

Zhou, Jiasi, Huiyun Xia, Haiwei Zuo, and Chintha Tellambura. 'Time Minimization for Health Monitoring Systems in Internet of Medical Things via Rate Splitting'. *IEEE Internet of Things Journal* 11, no. 4 (15 February 2024): 7186–97. https://doi.org/10.1109/jiot.2023.3315372.

Zhou, Kaiyang, Jingkang Yang, Chen Change Loy, and Ziwei Liu. 'Learning to Prompt for Vision-Language Models.' *International Journal of Computer Vision* 130, no. 9 (2022): 2337–2348. https://doi.org/10.1007/s11263-022-01626-9.

5 AI-Driven Health Coach for Diabetes Management

Mahalakshmi J., Balakrishnan C.,
Alisha Tharwani, and Seshathiri Dhanasekaran

5.1 INTRODUCTION

Rapid urbanization, shifting lifestyles, and genetic factors have contributed to a significant rise in diabetes prevalence in India, presenting substantial medical, social, and economic burdens across diverse populations. The International Diabetes Federation (IDF) reports that 463 million individuals aged 20–79 currently live with diabetes, while 374 million have impaired glucose tolerance. By 2045, this number is projected to rise to 693 million [1]. In India, often termed the "diabetes capital of the world," over 77 million individuals are presently under the influence of diabetes, with projections indicating that this number will escalate to 134 million by 2045. Diabetes specialists describe diabetes as a "gateway disease," warning that it is not simply about elevated blood sugar. It opens the door to heart disease, stroke, kidney failure, and a host of other complications, each progressively more severe. Recent advancements in digital health technologies, particularly in artificial intelligence, offer significant potential to enhance the delivery of diabetes care and help alleviate the growing financial burden of diabetes-related healthcare costs [2].

Proactive health management is essential to address the diabetes epidemic effectively. This includes regular blood glucose monitoring, adhering to a balanced diet, and incorporating physical activity into daily life. To aid these efforts, digital tools such as food-tracking apps, wearable devices, and continuous glucose monitors (CGMs) have become increasingly available. While these technologies provide valuable support, they often fail to meet the unique and diverse needs of individual patients. Many apps lack proper localization for regional diets, do not integrate seamlessly with healthcare systems, and offer generic insights that fall short of empowering users to make informed decisions. These limitations highlight the need for more tailored and comprehensive solutions to support individuals in managing their diabetes effectively.

The past five years have witnessed significant advancements in glucose monitoring, driven by the emergence of continuous glucose monitoring (CGM) systems, sophisticated automated analysis of novel glucose metrics, and the visualization of CGM data through ambulatory glucose profiles. Despite these advancements,

DOI: 10.1201/9781003476344-5

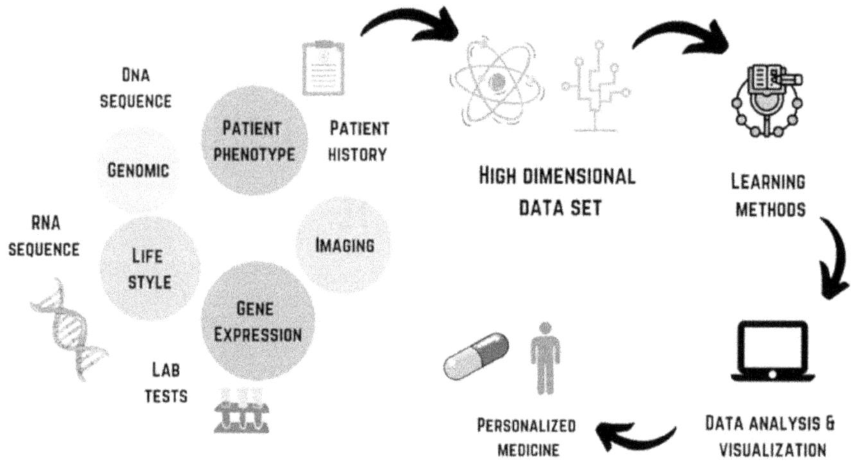

FIGURE 5.1 AI applications for the diabetics management (https://www.mdpi.com/BDCC/BDCC-07-00010/article_deploy/html/images/BDCC-07-00010-g001.png).

progress in identifying distinct subgroups of individuals with diabetes based on their unique glycemic patterns remains limited. Integrating behavioral and mental health data into these analyses has the potential to significantly improve subgroup identification and facilitate the development of precision medicine approaches tailored to individual patient needs [3].

Comprehensive diabetes care is essential, the basic AI Application for the diabetes management as depicted in Figure 5.1, as unmanaged diabetes can progress silently, leading to severe complications that early intervention could prevent. For individuals with diabetes (PwD), having access to tools that not only monitor their health but also deliver actionable insights is critical. Unfortunately, many current systems lack integration, leaving patients without clear guidance or meaningful data. Addressing these gaps requires a more personalized approach—one that prioritizes cultural relevance, offers real-time support, and takes individual needs into account to empower patients in managing their diabetes effectively.

Several authors have proposed a novel healthcare delivery model tailored to diabetes care in India. This model focuses on integrating key aspects of healthcare, including prevention, early diagnosis, and continuous management, to improve patient outcomes [4]. Nutrition and healthcare applications, such as the nutrition diet expert system (NDES), have shown exceptional performance in providing personalized dietary recommendations for diabetes management, achieving 96.48% accuracy, 0.98 precision, 0.96 recall, and an F1-score of 0.97. By optimizing dietary intake, insulin management, and lifestyle modifications, NDES plays a vital role in maintaining stable blood glucose levels, supporting healthy weight management, and enhancing overall outcomes in diabetes care [5].

This chapter aims to address existing limitations in diabetes care by introducing an innovative solution: AI-driven health coaches. These systems are designed to provide personalized and adaptive care, integrating real-time insights with cultural and regional considerations. By overcoming the shortcomings of current systems, AI-driven health coaches offer a seamless and integrated approach to diabetes management. Beyond a simple tool, this framework represents a paradigm shift toward dynamic, patient-centered care, where technology adapts to individual user needs, fostering long-term engagement and improved health outcomes. Through this chapter, we seek to highlight the potential of this approach and demonstrate how it can empower individuals with diabetes to manage their condition more effectively and confidently.

5.2 RELATED WORK

This section highlights the AI-based applications for the diabetes management along with their advantages and limitations over a period of time.

TABLE 5.1

S. No.	Year	Name of the Article	Technology/ Techniques Used	Insights	Reference
1	2022	Health care delivery model in India with relevance to diabetes care	Qualitative analysis, case studies	The paper emphasizes that diabetes represents a major public health challenge in India, driven by factors such as urbanization, lifestyle changes, and genetic predispositions. The growing prevalence of diabetes contributes to complications like cardiovascular diseases, kidney failure, and neuropathy, placing significant strain on the healthcare system	[4]
2	2024	Predictive model approach for enhancing diet management for diabetes patient through artificial intelligence	Random forest classifier	The authors of this research work developed the NDES, which employs the random forest classifier to provide personalized dietary recommendations for diabetes patients. This system is designed to optimize food intake, insulin management, and lifestyle changes—key factors in maintaining stable blood glucose levels	[5]

(Continued)

TABLE 5.1 (CONTINUED)

S. No.	Year	Name of the Article	Technology/ Techniques Used	Insights	Reference
3	2024	Artificial intelligence-driven transformations in diabetes care: a comprehensive literature review	Review article includes thorough state of art insights by using the PubMed database	The review underscores the transformative potential of AI in diabetes care, particularly in enhancing diagnosis, treatment, and disease management. The authors stress that AI can enable personalized treatment strategies for diabetes patients, allowing healthcare providers to customize interventions based on individual patient data, which could result in more effective disease management	[6]
4	2024	Novel adaptive AI-power insulin navigator for diabetes using machine learning	Adaptive AI algorithm and predictive analytics	The authors of the work concentrated on the incorporation of adaptive AI algorithms enables real-time adjustments to insulin dosages based on continuous glucose monitoring. This precision supports the maintenance of optimal blood glucose levels while minimizing the risks of hypoglycemia and hyperglycemia	[7]
5	2024	Utilizing artificial intelligence among patients with diabetes: a systematic review and meta-analysis	A comprehensive literature search was conducted across six electronic databases (Web of Science, Google Scholar, PubMed, Cochrane Library, EMBASE, and MEDLINE) to identify articles published between January 2019 and February 2024	This research emphasizes the need to widely adopt AI-powered solutions in healthcare settings to enhance patient outcomes and optimize treatment effectiveness. AI has the potential to significantly improve diabetes care through early detection and personalized lifestyle recommendation	[8]

(*Continued*)

TABLE 5.1 (CONTINUED)

S. No.	Year	Name of the Article	Technology/ Techniques Used	Insights	Reference
6	2024	Empowering patients with AI-driven personalized medicine: a paradigm shift in chronic disease management	This research emphasizes the use of AI to analyze vast datasets, enabling the identification of patterns that guide the development of personalized treatment plans. These regimens are tailored to individual patient characteristics, such as genetics, environment, and lifestyle	The authors discussed that the key outcome is the shift toward patient-centered care, where individuals are empowered to actively participate in their treatment journey, guided by personalized insights from AI. This enhanced engagement is crucial for improving adherence to treatment plans, particularly in the management of chronic conditions	[9]
7	2024	Artificial intelligence-based effective healthcare prediction system for diabetic patients	Min-max normalization, principal component analysis, tabu search-optimized bidirectional long short-term memory (TS-BiLSTM) model	This study showcases the TS-BiLSTM model, optimized with tabu search, achieving 95.72% accuracy in predicting healthcare outcomes for diabetic patients. The use of PCA for feature extraction enhanced performance by focusing on key variables, enabling precise predictions and valuable insights for diabetes management	[10]

5.3 DIABETICS

Diabetes mellitus is a long-term metabolic condition marked by persistent high blood sugar levels due to deficiencies in insulin production, insulin action, or a combination of both. Insulin, a hormone produced by the pancreas, is essential for maintaining blood glucose balance by enabling cells to absorb and use glucose effectively. In diabetes, either the pancreas produces insufficient insulin (Type 1 diabetes) or the body's cells become resistant to insulin's effects (Type 2 diabetes), resulting in chronically elevated blood sugar levels. Over time, this prolonged hyperglycemia can cause significant damage to various organs and systems.

5.3.1 Types of Diabetes

1. *Type 1 Diabetes:* Type 1 diabetes is an autoimmune disorder in which the body's immune system attacks and destroys the insulin-producing beta cells in the pancreas. It often develops during childhood or adolescence but can occur at any age. People with Type 1 diabetes require lifelong insulin therapy as their bodies are unable to produce insulin naturally.
2. *Type 2 Diabetes:* Type 2 diabetes is the most prevalent form, accounting for 90–95% of all cases. It occurs when the body either becomes resistant to insulin or the pancreas does not produce enough insulin to regulate blood sugar effectively. While it typically develops in adults, increasing rates of obesity and sedentary lifestyles have led to more cases among children and adolescents. Lifestyle changes, including a healthy diet, regular exercise, and weight management, can often prevent this form of diabetes.
3. *Gestational Diabetes:* Gestational diabetes occurs during pregnancy when the body cannot produce enough insulin to meet the needs of both the mother and the growing baby. Although it usually resolves after childbirth, women who experience gestational diabetes have a higher likelihood of developing Type 2 diabetes later in life. Additionally, babies born to mothers with gestational diabetes face an increased risk of obesity and developing Type 2 diabetes in the future.
4. *Prediabetes:* Prediabetes is a condition characterized by blood sugar levels that are elevated but not high enough to be diagnosed as Type 2 diabetes. It serves as an early warning, indicating an increased risk of developing Type 2 diabetes, heart disease, and stroke. However, adopting lifestyle changes such as a balanced diet and regular physical activity can reverse prediabetes and help prevent the progression to Type 2 diabetes.

5.3.2 Impact of Diabetes

Diabetes is often referred to as a "gateway disease" due to its extensive impact on overall health. When poorly controlled, diabetes greatly increases the likelihood of developing numerous severe complications:

- *Cardiovascular Complications:* High blood sugar accelerates atherosclerosis, raising the risk of heart attacks and strokes.
- *Kidney Disease:* Diabetic nephropathy can progress to kidney failure, often requiring dialysis.
- *Neuropathy:* Nerve damage caused by diabetes can affect the limbs, organs, and essential bodily functions.
- *Eye Disease:* Diabetic retinopathy may result in vision impairment or blindness.

- *Amputations:* Poor circulation and infections can lead to the necessity of limb amputations.

Beyond these direct complications, diabetes contributes to broader health concerns:

- *Increased Cancer Risk:* Chronic high blood sugar and insulin levels are associated with a greater risk of cancers such as liver, pancreatic, and colon cancers.
- *Cognitive Decline:* Persistent hyperglycemia can contribute to cognitive deterioration and a heightened risk of Alzheimer's disease.
- *Mental Health Challenges:* The continuous demands of diabetes management often lead to stress, anxiety, and depression.

Diabetes affects nearly every aspect of health, emphasizing the critical need for effective management to reduce its widespread and potentially life-threatening consequences.

5.3.3 Phases of Diabetes

5.3.3.1 Prevention: The Early Warning

Diabetes often begins with prediabetes, a stage marked by higher-than-normal blood sugar levels that have not yet reached the threshold for a diabetes diagnosis. This phase represents a crucial window for prevention. Unfortunately, many people remain unaware of how their lifestyle choices influence their diabetes risk until symptoms become evident. However, adopting proactive measures can effectively delay or even prevent the progression to diabetes. Preventive strategies focus on cultivating healthy lifestyle habits. Regular physical activity, such as walking, cycling, and so on can significantly improve insulin sensitivity. Engaging in at least 30 minutes of moderate-intensity exercise most days of the week has been shown to reduce the risk of developing Type 2 diabetes substantially. A balanced diet rich in whole grains, legumes, and vegetables plays a vital role in maintaining healthy blood sugar levels.

5.3.3.2 Phase 2: Diagnosis

A diabetes diagnosis can be initially overwhelming, but it also marks the beginning of a proactive journey toward effective management. Shifting from a potentially overlooked condition to one that demands consistent attention, diabetes management requires a commitment to daily care. This goes beyond simply reducing sugar intake; it involves a multifaceted approach encompassing a balanced diet, regular exercise, and, when necessary, medication. A well-balanced diet, rich in fiber from sources like lentils, chickpeas, spinach, and carrots, plays a crucial role in regulating blood sugar levels.

5.3.3.3 Phase 3: Control and Prevention of Complications

Effectively managing diabetes involves more than just controlling blood sugar—it also requires protecting overall health. Diabetes significantly increases the risk of heart disease, making it essential to prioritize heart-healthy choices. Incorporating foods rich in omega-3 fatty acids, such as fish and walnuts, while minimizing unhealthy fats supports cardiovascular health. Regular physical activity is equally important, as it helps reduce the risk of heart-related complications. Additionally, monitoring and maintaining healthy blood pressure levels is vital to safeguard the kidneys from potential damage caused by diabetes.

5.4 APPLICATIONS FOR MONITORING THE DIABETES: AN OVERVIEW

Managing diabetes demands consistent effort, including careful monitoring of blood sugar levels, diet, exercise, and medication adherence. Diabetes management apps have become essential tools in this process, offering real-time insights, personalized recommendations, and easy tracking of key health metrics. Popular options, including Glucose Buddy, HealthifyMe, MySugr, Glucomate, MyFitnessPal, Diabetolog, and Tidepool, are not specifically designed to "check" for diabetes but rather to assist in managing diabetes effectively. These are not the diagnosis applications, rather they focus on the metrics of blood sugar, weight, and dietary management.

The available apps for diabetes management are numerous, each offering different features and functionalities. To help you make an informed decision, we have compared the following apps based on critical parameters that contribute to an effective and personalized diabetes management experience.. The summary is given in the Figure 5.2, for varied applications.

5.4.1 Key Features of Diabetes Management Apps

- *Meal Input Flexibility:* Modern apps offer diverse meal input methods, including image scanning, barcode scanning, speech recognition, and food search, simplifying meal tracking, a crucial aspect of blood sugar control.
- *Accessibility and Cost:* The availability of a free version or affordable premium features is a significant factor. Many apps offer basic functionality for free, while advanced features may require a subscription.
- *Glucose Monitoring Integration:* Seamless integration with continuous glucose monitors (CGMs) or manual blood glucose meters ensures accurate and effective diabetes management.
- *User-Friendliness:* An intuitive and user-friendly interface is paramount, especially for older users or those less tech-savvy. Simplicity and clear navigation enhance accessibility for all.
- *Regional and Linguistic Support:* Support for regional cuisines and languages tailored to the user's location facilitates accurate food tracking and enhances app comprehension.

App Name	Meal Input Methods	Free of Charge	Glucose Monitoring	Ease of Use (30+ Years)	Regional Cuisine & Language Support	Voice & Chat Assistance	Weekly & Monthly Reports	Personalization
Glucose Buddy	✔ (Image, Barcode, Food Search)	✕	✔ (Manual Entry)	✔	✕ (Limited)	✕	✕	✔
HealthifyMe	✔ (Image, Barcode, Food Search)	✕	✕ (No direct glucose monitoring)	✔	✔ (Indian cuisines & multiple languages)	✔ (AI chat assistant)	✔	✔
mySugr	✕ (No Food Search)	✕	✔ (Manual Entry)	✔	✕	✕	✔	✔
Glucomate	✕ (No Food Search)	✕	✔ (Manual Entry)	✔	✕ (Limited)	✕	✕	✕
MyFitnessPal	✔ (Image, Barcode, Food Search)	✕	✕ (No direct glucose monitoring)	✔	✔ (Manual input for regional dishes)	✕	✔	✔
Diabetolog	✕ (No Food Search)	✕	✔ (Manual Entry)	✕	✕ (Limited)	✕	✕	✕
Tidepool	✕ (No Meal Input)	✔	✔ (Integrates with CGM/Glucose Meters)	✕	✕ (No cuisine support)	✕	✔	✕

FIGURE 5.2 Summary by app of features and functionalities.

- *AI and Voice Assistance:* Built-in AI or chatbot assistance provides personalized guidance and support. Voice commands further streamline navigation and data entry.
- *Comprehensive Reporting:* The ability to generate weekly and monthly reports summarizing glucose levels, meals, exercise, and overall progress is essential for ongoing monitoring and adjustments to diabetes care plans.
- *Personalized Recommendations:* Apps offering tailored recommendations, such as customized diet plans, exercise routines, and personalized glucose management advice, provide a highly individualized approach to diabetes management.

HealthifyMe is one of the most user-friendly apps, excelling in meal logging and offering features like food recognition, regional cuisine support, and multiple languages. However, its food recognition can be inconsistent, depending on the database used. Apps like Glucose Buddy and mySugr focus on glucose monitoring but require a premium subscription for additional features. Glucomate offers only glucose tracking with no meal logging, and Tidepool, while great for glucose device integration, is more complex and less accessible for general users. A common issue across many apps is the need for premium subscriptions to access critical features. MyFitnessPal, for example, limits advanced meal recognition tools to its premium version. Many

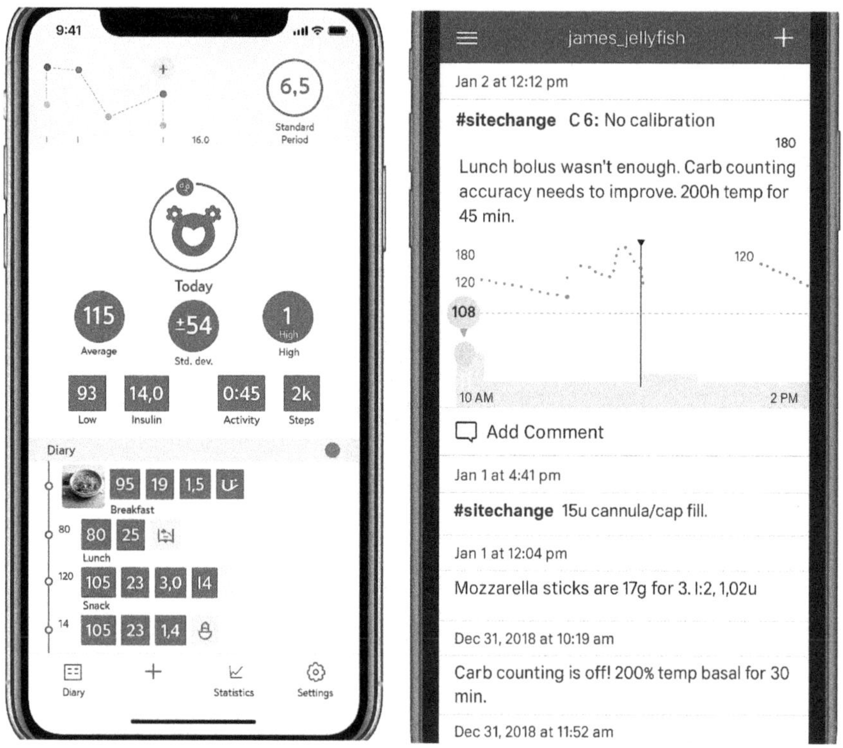

FIGURE 5.3 Reference images of Apps Mysugr, Glucosebuddy, and Tidepool.

apps also restrict meal logging to images taken directly through the app's camera, which can be frustrating. Despite these challenges, most apps offer user-friendly interfaces for easy navigation. However, apps like Diabetolog are limited by their lack of advanced features.

HealthifyMe stands out with its AI-powered chat assistant, providing personalized insights, making it a strong option for users seeking an all-in-one health tracker. A significant issue across apps is the variability in nutritional data, stemming from differences in food databases. While some apps offer community features and educational resources, none provide glycemic index information or detailed food preparation methods. No app offers a fully comprehensive solution, with gaps in features such as regional language support, personalized meal analysis, and integration of voice/chat assistance. This highlights the need for more inclusive and holistic platforms that cater to diverse users while ensuring accessibility. The reference images are given in the Figure 5.3 (a,b,c).

5.5 AI-DRIVEN FRAMEWORK FOR EMERGING DIABETES MANAGEMENT APPLICATIONS

The rising prevalence of diabetes in India, with millions affected, underscores the urgent need for innovative, accessible, and personalized solutions. Addressing the limitations of existing apps, this AI-driven framework focuses on bridging gaps in diabetes management while offering a user-friendly, inclusive, and efficient health management experience. The proposed app leverages artificial intelligence to redefine how individuals, particularly older adults, manage their conditions by incorporating advanced features and regional adaptability. This framework envisions a holistic solution that fills the gaps observed in existing applications, such as the inability to differentiate meal preparation methods (fried, steamed, boiled), limited regional language support, and fragmented user experiences. The AI health coach integrates diverse functionalities while maintaining simplicity, targeting users from varied linguistic and cultural backgrounds. The app incorporates several key features:

1. *AI-Powered Meal Analysis:* The app's meal scanner uses real-time photo analysis to identify food components, quantify nutritional values, and assess caloric content. It accounts for variations in preparation methods, like frying or steaming, to provide accurate nutritional insights. This feature surpasses existing apps by ensuring detailed and precise feedback on meal quality.
2. *Insulin and Medication Tracking:* Users can log their insulin doses and medication schedules, with the app monitoring irregularities and sending timely reminders. This proactive approach ensures adherence and reduces the risk of complications. If healthcare providers suggest changes in medication or dietary plans, the app adapts seamlessly, updating recommendations and reminders accordingly.
3. *Integration with Wearables and Real-Time Monitoring:* The app syncs with wearable devices to monitor vital health parameters, including glucose levels (via continuous glucose monitoring), heart rate, blood pressure, sleep patterns, and oxygen levels. These devices ensure real-time tracking and provide actionable insights, eliminating the need for manual data entry and ensuring users are always up-to-date with their health metrics.
4. *User-Friendly UI/UX and Dashboard:* The app is designed with simplicity in mind, akin to widely used platforms like WhatsApp and YouTube. Its intuitive interface ensures that even users aged 30–40+ can navigate it effortlessly. A dedicated dashboard provides an overview of health metrics, progress reports, and actionable recommendations, making diabetes management stress-free and straightforward.
5. *Weekly and Monthly Reporting:* The app automatically generates and emails detailed weekly and monthly health reports to users, healthcare providers, and guardians. These reports provide comprehensive insights into glucose levels, activity patterns, and adherence to dietary plans. This ensures stakeholders remain informed and can take timely action if needed.

6. *Voice and Chat Assistance:* The app offers voice and chatbot support in multiple Indian languages, guiding users through health-related queries, meal logging, and activity tracking. This feature is especially beneficial for older adults and individuals less comfortable with technology, ensuring they can easily engage with the app.

The proposed diabetes management framework as depicted in Figure 5.4 is designed with a strong focus on *localization*, *regional cuisine support*, and *language*

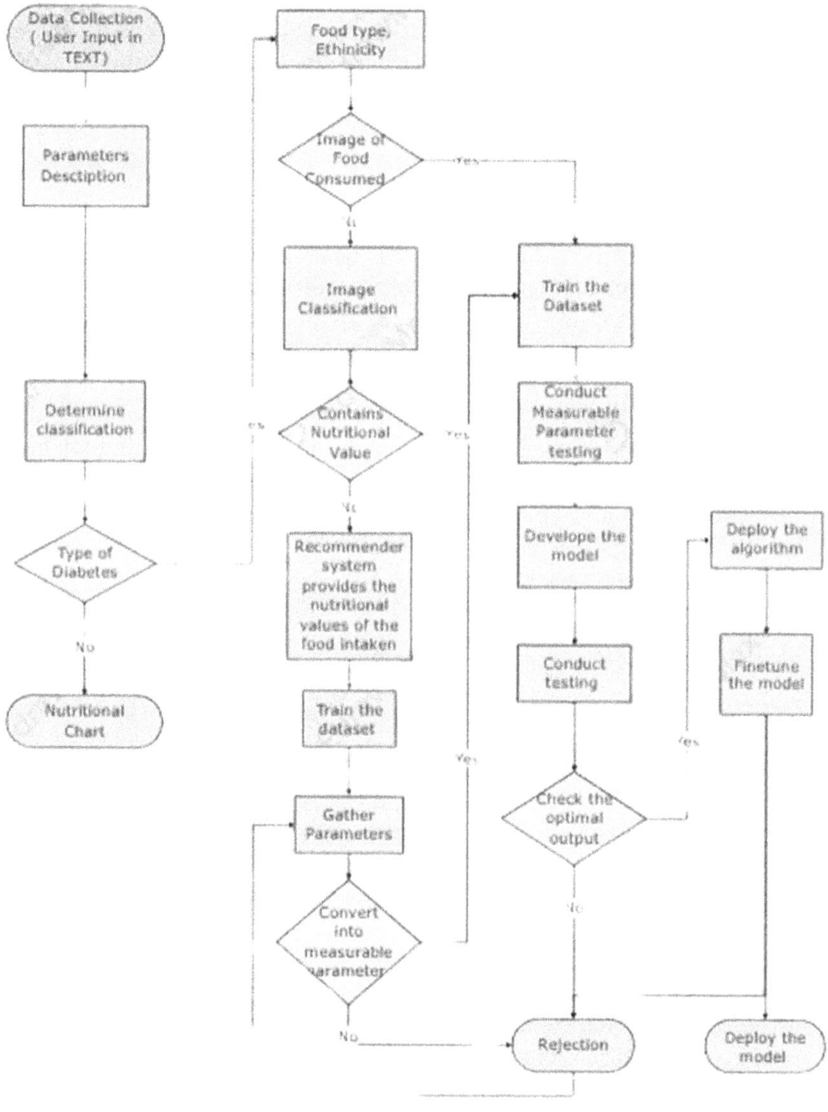

FIGURE 5.4 Proposed framework for meal scanner.

assistance, ensuring accessibility and effectiveness for diverse user groups. The system is built to handle a wide range of languages and food types, making it adaptable to the cultural and dietary needs of users across different regions. Here is a more detailed breakdown of the workflow with a focus on language, cuisine, and voice/chat assistance:

1. **User Onboarding and Profile Setup**

During the initial onboarding process, users are prompted to select their *preferred language* from a wide range of options. The system also takes into account the user's *dietary preferences* (vegetarian, non-vegetarian) and *regional food habits*. This allows the framework to personalize meal suggestions and health tips based on the user's local context.

2. **Glucose Monitoring Integration**

Once the profile is set, users can sync their glucose monitoring devices (CGMs or manual glucose meters). The real-time glucose data is processed and displayed in the app. The app supports multiple languages for displaying glucose data, making it easier for non-English speakers to understand their health status. The system also adapts the data display to the local context to improve understanding (e.g., units of measurement like mg/dL or mmol/L).

5.5.1 Standard Equation for Blood Glucose Conversion

The measurement and interpretation of blood glucose levels are fundamental to effective diabetes management. Blood glucose is typically expressed in two units: milligrams per deciliter (mg/dL), commonly used in the United States, and millimoles per liter (mmol/L), widely adopted in Europe and other regions. To ensure consistency and compatibility across devices and platforms, a standardized equation is used to convert between these units. This conversion is crucial for applications and devices aiming to serve a global audience.

Conversion Formula

The relationship between mg/dl and mmol/L is expressed mathematically as follows:

mmol/L=mg/dL18\text{mmol/L} = \frac{\text{mg/dL}}{18}mmol/L=18mg/dL

Factor of 18: The conversion factor (18) arises from the molecular weight of glucose ($C_6H_{12}O_6$), which is approximately 180 g/mol, and the need to normalize it per liter and milligrams. This standard is internationally recognized and validated by leading health organizations and device manufacturers.

Application: Devices such as Apple Health, Dexcom CGMs, and other major health platforms rely on this equation to display glucose readings accurately, irrespective of the user's location or preferred unit of measurement. This conversion ensures that users and healthcare providers can interpret glucose data consistently, facilitating better decision-making and management of diabetes.

Example Calculations 1. If a device records a glucose level of 100 mg/dL, the equivalent in mmol/L is calculated as follows:

mmol/L=10018≈5.56\text{mmol/L} = \frac{100}{18}
approx 5.56mmol/L=18100 ≈5.56 2.

Conversely, a reading of 6 mmol/L can be converted to mg/dL as follows: mg/dL=6×18=108\text{mg/dL} = 6 \times 18 = 108mg/dL=6×18=10

3. **Meal Logging and Analysis: Regional Cuisine and Language Support**

Meal input is a critical component of managing diabetes, and the framework excels in this area by offering various ways to log meals, each with *local language support*:

- *Image Scanning:* Users can take pictures of their meals, and the app uses *image recognition technology* to identify the food. The recognition engine has been trained to understand *regional cuisines* and provides nutritional information based on locally available foods. Users can log meals in their *preferred language*, ensuring the experience feels personalized and familiar.
- *Barcode Scanning:* For packaged foods, users can scan the barcode, and the app fetches the nutritional data in the user's chosen language. The app supports popular regional products and includes local food packaging from diverse regions.
- *Food Search:* The app offers a comprehensive *food database* with entries for traditional foods across various cultures and regions. Users can search for specific items using local terms (e.g., "idli" instead of "steamed rice cakes"), and the app will provide accurate nutritional analysis in the selected language.
- *Speech Input:* Users can log meals verbally through *speech recognition technology*. This functionality allows users to speak in their regional language and log their meals hands-free. The app then processes the speech input and converts it into text, making it easier for users to log their meals without having to type.

These features ensure that users from diverse linguistic backgrounds can easily navigate and use the app, with *regional language support* for both the interface and meal tracking. The app ensures that the food's nutritional details are presented in a way that aligns with the user's cultural context.

4. **Exercise Tracking and Suggestions**

The framework not only tracks meals but also provides *exercise suggestions* based on the user's activity levels and glucose trends. *Voice commands* can be used to log physical activity, and the system supports local languages for providing exercise instructions and tips.

5. **AI-Powered Insights and Recommendations**

Using *AI and machine learning*, the framework analyzes collected data from glucose levels, meals, and exercise to offer actionable insights. These insights are tailored to the user's specific needs, health goals, and regional dietary habits. For example, the app might suggest switching from *white rice* to *brown rice* based on glucose patterns or recommend adding more *fiber-rich local vegetables* to meals.

6. **Voice and Chat Assistance**

The *voice assistant* and *chatbot* capabilities are integrated into the framework to offer personalized support. The voice assistant can be activated in the user's chosen language, making it easier to interact with the app without needing to navigate complex menus.

7. **Data Sharing and Collaboration with Healthcare Providers**

The app facilitates *data sharing* with healthcare providers, enabling a *collaborative approach* to diabetes management. Users can send their glucose data, meal logs, and activity reports to their healthcare providers in the app's chosen language. This makes it easier for doctors to review patient data and adjust treatment plans accordingly. The system also supports *real-time chat* with healthcare providers, where users can receive advice and suggestions in their preferred language.

Continuous Learning and Adaptation

As the user interacts with the app, the system *learns and adapts* to their preferences and health trends. The AI constantly adjusts meal suggestions, exercise recommendations, and health insights based on the user's data. The system also takes cultural preferences into account, refining its understanding of regional foods, dietary habits, and language nuances over time.

5.7 CONCLUSION

While the current diabetes management tools have made significant strides in personalization, language support, and regional cuisine integration, the field continues to evolve. As technology advances, we can expect even more refined tools that will improve the accuracy and effectiveness of these apps. One promising area is the integration of wearables. Future apps will likely work seamlessly with smartwatches, continuous glucose monitors (CGMs), and fitness trackers, providing real-time data on blood sugar levels, physical activity, and sleep patterns.

This integration will allow for more precise diabetes management and offer early warnings for potential health issues, enabling proactive interventions. For instance, wearables could monitor blood sugar levels and automatically adjust insulin doses, offering a hands-off experience for users. Additionally, as machine learning and artificial intelligence improve, apps will become even smarter, offering highly personalized recommendations. By analyzing real-time data on a user's lifestyle, medical history, and preferences, future systems will not only react to past data but also predict future health trends. This predictive capability will allow for more accurate suggestions regarding diet, exercise, and blood sugar management, integrating diabetes care into daily life with less reliance on manual input.

Alongside advancements in wearables, data privacy and security will remain a priority, especially as these apps handle sensitive health information. The use of blockchain and advanced encryption technologies may play a significant role in protecting this data, ensuring users feel confident sharing it with healthcare providers and other stakeholders. As the ecosystem of healthcare apps, wearables, and data sharing expands, ensuring interoperability and seamless communication across platforms will be key to unlocking the full potential of future diabetes management technologies.

REFERENCES

1. Ellahham, S. MD. (2020, August). Artificial intelligence: The future for diabetes care. *The American Journal of Medicine,* 133(8). https://doi.org/10.1016/j.amjmed.2020.03.033
2. Guan, Z., Li, H., et al. (2023). Artificial intelligence in diabetes management: Advancements, opportunities, and challenges. *Cell Reports Medicine,* 4(10). https://doi.org/10.1016/j.xcrm.2023.101213.
3. Hermanns, N., Ehrmann, D., Shapira, A., et al. (2022). Coordination of glucose monitoring, self-care behaviour and mental health: Achieving precision monitoring in diabetes. *Diabetologia,* 65, 1883–1894. https://doi.org/10.1007/s00125-022-05685-7
4. Das, A. K., Saboo, B., Maheshwari, A., Nair, M. V., Banerjee, S., C., B. V., Prasobh, S. P., Ranjit Mohan, A., Potty, V. S., & Kesavadev, J. (2022). Health care delivery model in India with relevance to diabetes care. *Heliyon,* 8(10), e10904. https://doi.org/10.1016/j.heliyon.2022.e10904.
5. Singh Bhadouria, A., & Ahirwar, A. (2024). Predictive model approach for enhancing diet management for diabetes patients through artificial intelligence. In *Advances in medical technologies and clinical practice* (pp. 335–366). https://doi.org/10.4018/979-8-3693-8990-4.ch015.
6. Iftikhar, M., Saqib, M., Qayyum, S. N., Asmat, R., Mumtaz, H., Rehan, M., Ullah, I., Ud-Din, I., Noori, S., Khan, M., Rehman, E., & Ejaz, Z. (2024). Artificial intelligence-driven transformations in diabetes care: A comprehensive literature review. *Annals of Medicine and Surgery.* https://doi.org/10.1097/ms9.0000000000002369.
7. Deekshith, A. (2024). Novel adaptive ai-power insulin navigator for diabetes using machine learning. *Deleted Journal,* 11(8), 57–74. https://doi.org/10.26662/ijiert.v11i8.pp57-74.

8. Alhalafi, A., Alqahtani, S. M., Alqarni, N. A., Aljuaid, A. T., Aljaber, G. T., Alshahrani, L. M., Mushait, H., & Nandi, P. A. (2024). Utilizing artificial intelligence among patients with diabetes: A systematic review and meta-analysis. *Cureus*. https://doi.org/10.7759/cureus.58713.
9. Ananya, S. (2024). Empowering patients with ai-driven personalized medicine: A paradigm shift in chronic disease management. *International Journal of Advanced Research*. https://doi.org/10.21474/ijar01/19340.
10. Ramasamy, M., Acharjya, K., Singh, Y., & Gupta, R. (2024). Artificial intelligence-based effective healthcare prediction system for diabetic patients. *Multidisciplinary Science Journal,* 6, 2024ss0303. https://doi.org/10.31893/multiscience.2024ss0303

6 An Enhancement of Security System Using Curve-Based Cryptosystem with Decentralized Scalable Group Key Agreement for IoMT

Kavitha S., Alphonse P.J.A., and Muthu Ramachandran

6.1 INTRODUCTION

IoT encompasses various subgroups, with Internet of Medical Things (IoMT) being important, which is concerned with connectivity and communication between objects, or things. IoMT is the combination of medical professionals, patients, and equipment, like wearables, hospital equipment, and diagnostic tools. Internet access is implemented at hospitals to improve patient care through IoMT.

Here is the representation of IoMT used for patient care:

- Patient with chronic diseases and long-term conditions has been monitored using remote patient monitoring.
- Monitoring the specified locations of hospitalized patients and their prescription of medicine, as well as linking the routes taken by ambulances to healthcare providers. In the period of COVID 19 pandemic, as a means to reduce patients traveling to healthcare facilities and to alleviate the pressure on overworked hospitals and other medical facilities
- Medical employees receive updates on the number of medical supplies and equipment present on stock as well as their location when RFID tags are affixed to these items.

DOI: 10.1201/9781003476344-6

6.1.1 Evolution of IoMT

IoMT has evolved alongside advancements in IoT, cloud computing, and artificial intelligence (AI). Initially, medical devices operated in isolation, requiring manual data collection and analysis. With the advent of wireless technologies, these devices have become interconnected, enabling remote patient monitoring and telemedicine. IoMT systems now integrate AI to process vast datasets, providing predictive insights and personalized healthcare solutions.

6.1.2 Major Components of IoMT

1. *Wearable Devices:* Smartwatches, fitness trackers, and biosensors monitor vital signs and physical activity in real time.
2. *Medical Equipment:* Devices like infusion pumps, ventilators, and imaging systems are IoT-enabled for real-time data access and management.
3. *Communication Networks:* IoMT relies on Bluetooth, Wi-Fi, and 5G technologies to ensure seamless connectivity.
4. *Data Storage and Processing Platforms:* Cloud and edge computing facilitate secure data storage and analysis.
5. *Healthcare Applications:* These include electronic health records (EHRs), telemedicine platforms, and mobile apps for patient engagement.

6.1.3 Use Cases of IoMT

- *Remote Patient Monitoring (RPM):* Devices monitor patients with chronic diseases, reducing hospital visits and enabling early intervention.
- *Telemedicine:* IoMT supports virtual consultations, particularly valuable in rural or underserved regions.
- *Smart Hospitals:* IoMT optimizes resource management, such as tracking medical equipment with RFID tags and automating inventory management.
- *Emergency Response:* Ambulances equipped with IoMT enable real-time data sharing with hospitals, improving preparedness.

6.1.4 Challenges in IoMT

1. *Interoperability:* Diverse IoMT devices and systems often lack standardization, complicating integration.
2. *Cybersecurity Risks:* IoMT devices are prone to vulnerabilities like unauthorized data access, ransomware, and system breaches.
3. *Ethical Concerns:* Issues of data privacy, informed consent, and bias in AI algorithms must be addressed Xin (2015).

One of the major difficulties in IoMT is weak security. Most of the IoMT devices were not configured with security in mind, which makes them vulnerable to compromise. The IoMT has a variety of security challenges that require comprehensive ways to avoid potential complications. Attackers may take advantage of the security flaws in IoMT devices to obtain unauthorized access to private information or interfere with normal operation of the device. Concerns of patient privacy and security against unauthorized access are brought up by the easy transfer of patient data across linked medical devices. It can be difficult to guarantee smooth communication and compatibility across various IoMT devices, which could result in security flaws. Cyberattacks against healthcare systems have increased noticeably, which raises the dangers of patient data disclosure, hospital information leakage, and service interruptions. IoMT needs efficient security system since security breach in a medical network can quite literally become a matter of losing lives.

This chapter identifies the security vulnerabilities and proposes various innovative solutions to handle the security threats. By adopting a hybrid approach, the group supports both key generation and the establishment of a novel curve-based security framework.

6.1.5 System Architecture of IoMT

- Layers such as devices (sensors, wearables), communication networks, cloud/edge computing, and applications.
- Highlight security protocols (e.g., AES, ECC) at each layer.

Figure 6.1 shows the mindmap diagram. It illustrates the layered architecture of IoMT, which integrates smart devices, networks, and cloud computing for efficient healthcare delivery. At the base, devices like sensors (e.g., heart rate monitors) and wearables (e.g., fitness trackers) collect real-time health data. These devices communicate through networks like Bluetooth, Wi-Fi, or cellular technology to transmit data securely to cloud or edge servers. Cloud-edge computing processes and stores this data, enabling scalable and low-latency access. Finally, applications such as patient monitoring and health analytics utilize this information for actionable insights. Stallings (2017).

Security is paramount in IoMT. For example, AES (Advanced Encryption Standard) encrypts device data, ensuring confidentiality, while ECC (Elliptic Curve Cryptography) secures key exchanges, protecting against attacks. Adedeji and Famoriji (2014). These protocols maintain privacy even during data transmission and processing.

6.2 PROPOSED WORK

6.2.1 Hybrid Cryptographic Algorithm for IoT Medical Things

The hybrid cryptosystem includes Diffie–Hellman (DH) and Advanced Encryption Standard 128 bit (AES) algorithm that has been implemented along the twisted Hessian curve (HC) cryptosystem. The algorithms are represented in two phases of symmetric and asymmetric cryptographic mechanism called AES_HC and DH_HC. HC is preferred over ECC, as it requires less calculation (Kavitha et al., 2019).

TABLE 6.1
Survey and Critical Evaluation of Cryptographic Approaches in IoMT Security

Approach	Description	Strengths	Weaknesses	Applications
Elliptic curve cryptography (ECC)	Lightweight cryptography using elliptic curves for secure key exchange	High security at low computational cost	Vulnerable to quantum attacks	Remote patient monitoring, device pairing
Advanced encryption standard (AES)	Symmetric encryption algorithm for data protection	High efficiency for bulk data encryption	Key distribution is challenging	Data storage in smart hospitals
Hybrid cryptosystem (AES-DH)	Combines AES and Diffie–Hellman for confidentiality and secure key exchange	Reduces key generation overhead	Complex implementation in resource-limited devices	Real-time monitoring systems
Hyper-elliptic curve cryptography (HECC)	Generalization of ECC with higher genus curves for enhanced security	Smaller key sizes for equal security levels	Computationally intensive for large data	Encrypted communication in IoMT networks
RSA with Burnside curve	Employs novel curves for RSA, enhancing security with smaller key sizes	High resistance to subgroup attacks	Requires further optimization for scalability	Secure storage and transmission of patient records

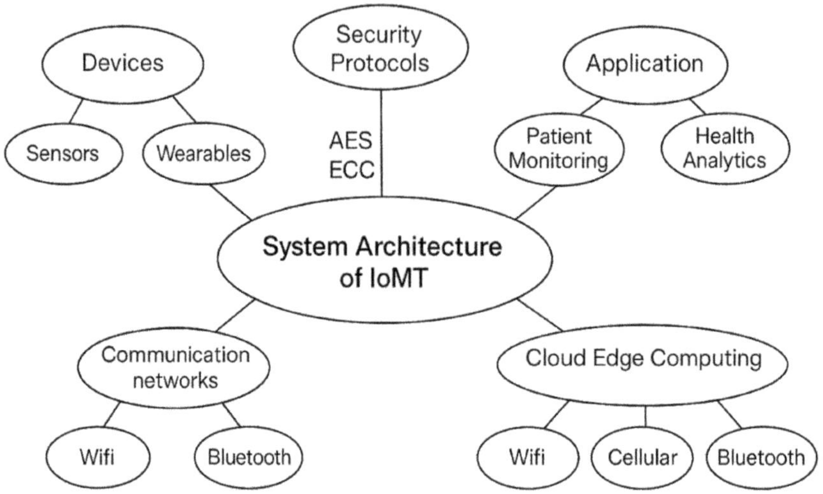

FIGURE 6.1 System architecture of IoMT.

6.2.1.1 Cryptographic Protocol Flow

Figure 6.2 illustrates a hybrid cryptosystem combining *AES* (symmetric encryption) with Diffie–Hellman (DH) (asymmetric key exchange).

1. The system starts by generating an *AES session key* for encrypting sensitive IoMT data like ECG readings.
2. A secure *DH key exchange* distributes this key to a cloud server.
3. IoMT data is encrypted with AES and transmitted alongside the key.
4. The cloud decrypts the data using the DH key, ensuring both speed and security.

For example, in a wearable glucose monitor, AES encrypts glucose level data for quick transmission, while DH ensures that only authorized cloud servers can decrypt it (Bernstein et al., 2008; Bernstein and Lange, 2014). This hybrid approach balances performance and security.

The HC is used to translate the text message into coordinates of x, y, which are then fed into AES_HC. This procedure eliminates known plain text attack. Unlike AES 128 bit, which processes in rounds, DH key exchange and its variant Hessian curve-based Diffie–Hellman (DH_HC) generate the shared key all at once, it reduces the computational cost of the key generation technique. It is considered as to the benefit of the DH_HC algorithm that is a significantly reduced computation of AES key generation. An asymmetric algorithm perceives security hold as symmetric key. Thus, the asymmetric key exchange coupled with symmetric DH_HC algorithm is proposed. The AES_HC algorithm enhances the security measurement by privacy and truthfulness, DH_HC handles the key exchange process. This procedure is used

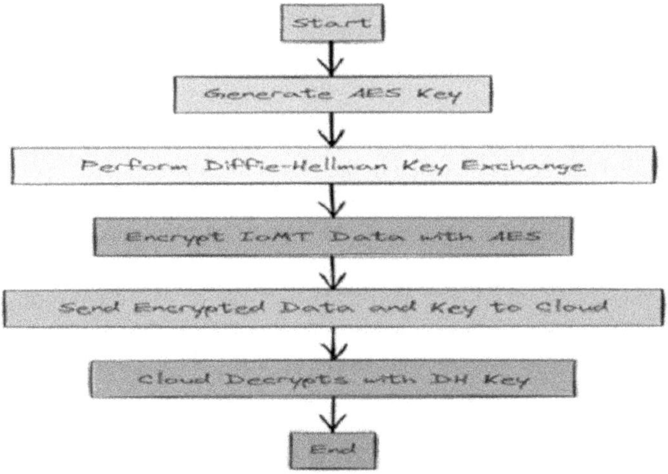

FIGURE 6.2 A flowchart illustrating the use of a hybrid cryptosystem that combines AES and Diffie–Hellman for encrypting and decrypting IoMT data.

to eliminate the drawback of the HMAC-based key derivation function (HKDF) (Mathur et al., 2017) .

The field K of an affine coordinate system is represented in the twisted Hessian curve:

$$HC : l\ ax^3 + y^3 + 1 = dxy \tag{6.1}$$

Additive and doubling operations are computed for scalar multiplication of HC. Here a variable assigned as 1, d is in Field K, derives equation (6.1).

Let $p = (x_1, y_1)$ and $q = (x_2, y_2)$, then

$r = p + q = (x_3, y_3)$ is derived by the succeeding equations:

$$x_3 = \frac{x_1 - y_1 * x_2 * y_2}{a * x_1 * y_1 * x_2^2 - y_2} \tag{6.2}$$

$$y_3 = \frac{y_1 * y_2^2 - a * x_1^2 * x_2}{a * x_1 * y_1 * x_2^2 - y_2} \tag{6.3}$$

Let $p = (x, y)$, compute $2p$ as (x_3, y_3)

$$x_3 = \frac{x - y^3 * x}{a * y * x^3 - y} \tag{6.4}$$

$$y_3 = \frac{y^3 - a * x^3}{a * y * x^3 - y} \tag{6.5}$$

The three phases of proposed hybrid algorithm (AES_DH) HC are implemented by the following procedure (Kavitha et al., 2019).

Phase I: The message is embedded on the Hessian curve which is considered as the X-axis and coordinates.

Phase II: DH_HC algorithm is used to generate private and public keys.

Phase III: Private key is included in the first round of AES_HC.

Figures 6.3 and 6.4 show that AES_HC and DH_HC achieve minimum execution times than their standard counter part, AES and DH (Alphonse and Reddy, 2019; Kavitha et al., 2019).

The comparison of mentioned algorithms is made by execution time, block size, and key size. The hybrid algorithm executes faster than the individual algorithms (Bernstein et al., 2008; Adedeji and Famoriji, 2014; Thangavelu and Vijaykumar, 2016; Xin, 2015).

The average data rate (AVG_R) is calculated through (AES_DH) HC algorithm by providing various data sizes in kb/s and data value in kb/s:

$$AVG_R = \frac{1}{tb_i} \sum_{i=1}^{tb} \frac{m}{t_i} \tag{6.6}$$

$$T_P = \frac{N_b}{T} \tag{6.7}$$

Here total number of plain texts are noted in tb, message is represented by m in kb, and t_i is the notation of time in seconds. Throughput is determining how long an algorithm takes to execute, which is used to assess an algorithm's performance. In Eq. (6.7), N_b is the total amount of text message expressed in kb and T is the time expressed in seconds; this is required to finish the encryption and decryption procedures. The execution timings for (AES_DH) HC encryption and decryption are compared with those of Adedeji and Famoriji (2014).

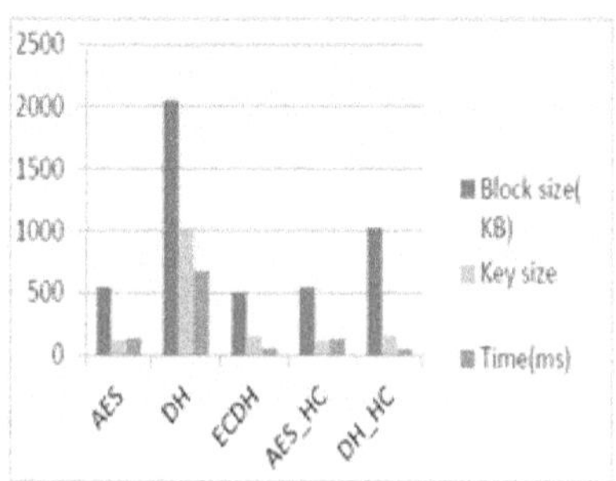

FIGURE 6.3 Different algorithms execution time.

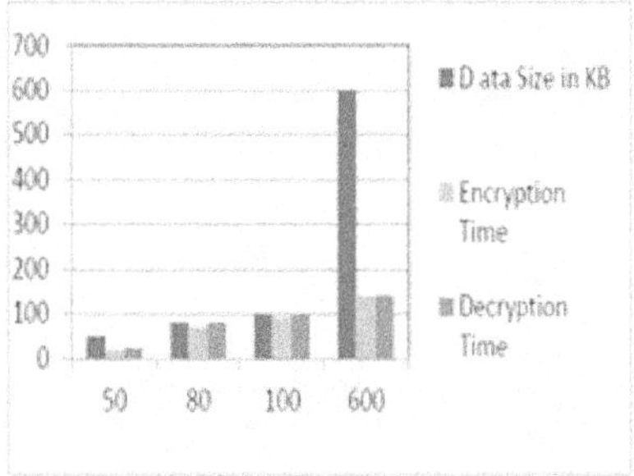

FIGURE 6.4 Execution time for encryption and decryption.

6.2.2 Scalable Group Key Agreement Scheme for Hierarchical Structure–Based IoT Medical Things

Due to the risk of malwares or unauthorized users exploiting vulnerabilities on the group communication, group members' medical data–based communications should always be safe. To propose an approach, keep in mind that decentralized scalable group key agreement leads to accuracy of the group communication. Alphonse and Reddy (2019) proposed a method for group key generation, where there is no central key management control system. When communicating with other groups as well as within subgroups, each member of the group is considered as having equal privilege and the ability to generate the group key (Veltri et al., 2013).

Thus, decentralized group structure has been eliminating single-point failure in group key agreement (Figure 6.5). In this structure, each subgroup is called sg_i, and it consists of sg_{im-2} phases. In each phase, three members participate in order to generate partial keys. It has transferred over adjacent nodes to the last subgroup member, who serves as each subgroup's initiator and compound of partial keys are used to produce group key. sg_{im} creates the key with the combination of partial keys with private keys, which may be either unicast or multicast to subgroup sg_i.

The encrypted message represented by $sg_i p_i x_n$, which is partial key with private key of their own. sg_i subgroup partial keys are shown by $sg_1 p_1 x_1 \cdots sg_i p_i x_n$. It originates from $hcds(m_j)$, $t_i, su_i m_j$, where $hcds(m_i)$ is hash function of jth message, $su_i m_j$ denotes ith member and jth text message, and t_i is the power of primitive root computation with mod operation. The group members are named by the way of $sg_{im} = [sg_{im}, sg_{im-1}, sg_{im-2}, sg_{im+1}, sg_{im+2}, \ldots, sg_{im+n}, \ldots, sg_{im-n}]$

where $i = 1, 2, \ldots, n$.

The dynamic group key refreshment has two motivations: whenever a new member join or leave the subgroup, the group key agreement may be refreshed. When a new member request to join sg_i, it comes to know the members of the subgroup who needs to refresh key, which can be identified by virtual subnet ID. The transferred partial key along with virtual subnet ID (VSID) is used to find the corresponding sg_i needed for rekeying process and update group key based on derivation method.

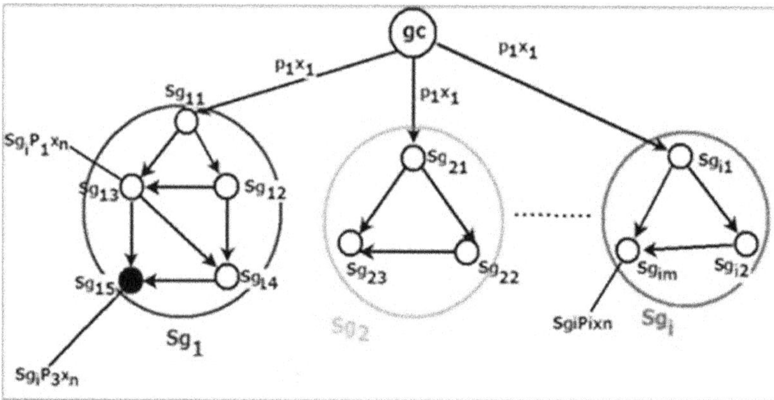

FIGURE 6.5 Decentralized group key structure–based IoMT (Kavitha and Alphonse, 2019)

$new(sg_ip_ix_j) = p_ix_i = (hcds(m_i), t, su_im_i)$, which is multicast to members, is encrypted by the previous key $sg_ip_ix_n$. Here $(sg_ip_ix_n)$j is the updated version of $sg_ip_ix_n$ in sg_i, it is unicast to newly join member through secure channel. Altogether, sg_i group member update their partial keys through changing of (private key) random number. Moreover, leaving member request to initiator sg_i, who has broadcast to all in the form of sign(sg_{im}, $(leave(sg_i)$. After verification, rekeying process is computed by changing the private key $sg_ip_ix_n$ on their own; further generation of partial key is distributed to neighbor nodes. In the rekeying process, gc select the random integer $z \in [1 > z < p - 1]$ and perform the partial key $sg_ip_ix_n$ generation, which is broadcast to all first member of sgs. Here sg_i who receives the message has computed $sg_ip_ix_n$:

$$
\begin{aligned}
sg_ip_ix_n &= En(hcds(m_i), t_i, su_im_j) \\
&= En(p_1x_1, \ldots, p_1x_n, p_2x_1, \ldots, p_2x_n, \ldots, p_ix_1, \ldots, p_ix_n)
\end{aligned}
$$

$sg_ip_ix_n$ generation is done with the random selection of private keys $x_1, x_2, \ldots, x_n$.

The partial key generation process compute by number of phases in sg_i, every p_ix_n *is* transferred to the corresponding members in a sg_i. The number of phases in each sg_i is sg_{im-2} and in transfer partial keys sg_{im+1} times, which is total number of transmissions over group. Let jn denote joining member broadcast message. The joining operation communication cost has been defined by $sg_{im+1}jn$.

$$
gc = \sum_{i,m=1}^{n} sg_{im+1} * jn \tag{6.8}
$$

ln denotes the board-casting message of leaving operation to all. The sg_{im+1} times transfer the partial keys in sg_{im-2} phases. The communication cost of the leaving member operation in this method is defined by

$$
gc = \sum_{i,m=1}^{n} sg_{im+1} * \ln \tag{6.9}
$$

Here rekeying process for leaving and joining member in the group

of sg_i is considered. The computation of communication cost for rekeying process can be defined as aggregate of two processes of joining and leaving members in the group:

$$gc = \sum_{i,m=1}^{n} sg_{im+1} * (jn + \ln) \tag{6.10}$$

In the leaving/joining process, partial key alone is transmitted securely. Hence, proposed method efficiently reduces the communication cost for group key generation.

6.2.3 Group Key Settlement for IoMT through Hyperelliptic Curve Cryptosystem

The desired level of security system is currently satisfied by cryptographic transformations on elliptic curves due to growing technological capability in IoMT networks and the development of cryptanalysis techniques. Hyperelliptic Curve Cryptography (HECC), replaces elliptic curve cryptography, which may lead to an increase in the stability of the security system.

Consider the value p is the prime number. In the finite field fp of hyperelliptic curve Hc of genus >2 is used to in the following equation:

$$Hc\colon y^2 + h(x)y = f(x) \tag{6.11}$$

deg(f) = 2g+1 $deg(h) \leq g$, f *monic* polynomial fulfils the equation $y^2 + h(x)\, y = f(x)$ and the partial derivative equation $2y + h(x) = 0$ & $h(x)y - f(x) = 0$. Additionally, the curve Hc has a set of K-rational points that are non-singular.

The hyperelliptic curves Hc and g, which have a reduced divisor of large prime number in $J(fp)$, are employed for authentication. The divisor scalar multiplication of D is denoted as kg, multiplied by integer k and [.] E denotes an aligning from $J(f_p)$ to $Z_p 2g$. Message signature generation procedure is performed by the selection of Map $f(r, m, kg)$, then selected random integer is applied to solve r_i, s_i from the equation $F(r, m, kg) = 0$. The solution of (r_i, s_i) fulfilled with the state $s_i r_i \equiv 0$. Signature verification process performed by divisor scalar multiplication over Hc is then signature verified whether it has been approved or denied.

The mentioned equation is used to verify the signature:

$$R = s_{i-1} h(m_i) G + s_{i-1} r_i n \tag{6.12}$$
$$F\,(r, m, o^{-1})\,(r, s, m)\,(-t\,(r, s, m)\,n) - q\,(r, s.m)g) = 0$$

Signature (ri, si) is message m, validity is guaranteed. Hc plays major role in an IoT which includes context, computational capacity, storage, and data transfer rate are performed on a better level than ECC Bernstein and Lange (2014). By using the HcElgamal (HcElg) algorithm, protected group communication has enabled through generalized scalable group key agreement protocol. HcDSA ensure authentication and security, that handles the known possible attacks in efficiently. Moreover,

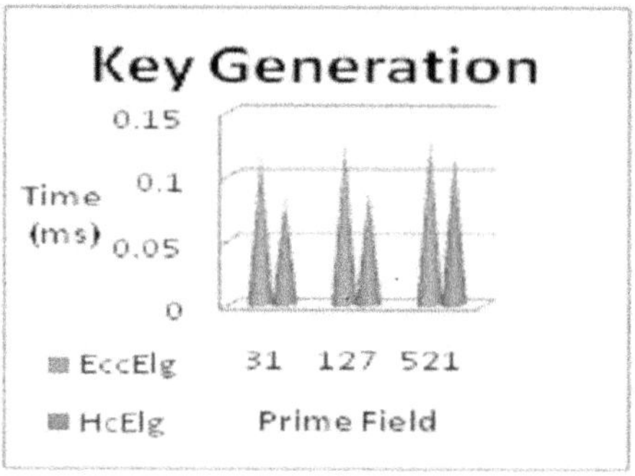

FIGURE 6.6 EccElg and HcElg key generation.

effectiveness of HcDSA is demonstrated by addition and doubling arithmetic operations and it also proves security is equivalent to 1024 bit, much stronger than 160 bit DSA. This method extracts efficiency and secure system for IoMT as Jaiswal and Tripathi (2017). Figures 6.6, 6.7, and 6.8 show the algorithm execution time of HcElg and EcElg (Kavitha et al., 2019; Kavitha and Alphonse, 2019). The algorithm execution times are analyzed for key generation, encryption, and decryption across different prime fields. This leads one to the conclusion that HcElg executes faster than EcElg (Kavitha et al., 2019).

6.2.4 Implementation of Genus 2 Hyperelliptic Curve Cryptosystem

The proposed cryptosystem produces efficient way of implementation on the Jacobin of HEC that proves an efficiency of identity authentication by digital signature, key generation by Diffie–Hellman, and finally through encryption/decryption of AES. The HEC-based cryptosystem is denoted as *HC(DSADH_AES)*. The hyperelliptic curve $HC = x^5 + x^3 + 1$ is used to publicly known standard parameters. The encapsulated process of message covered through hyperelliptic curve is based on AES_{128}- 10 round process algorithm. The major part of AES key generation 128 bit key –10

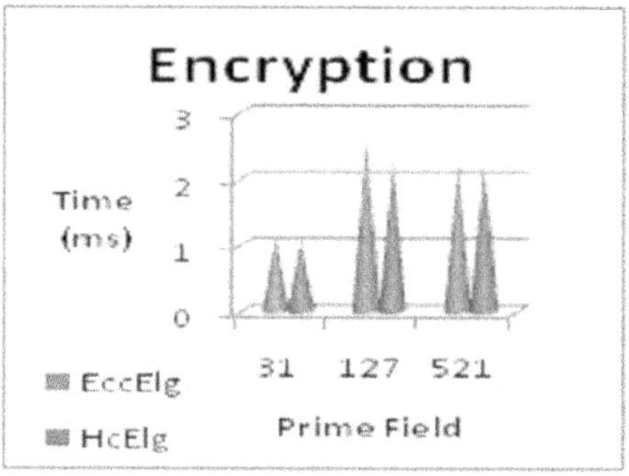

FIGURE 6.7 Encryption time – EccElg and HcElg.

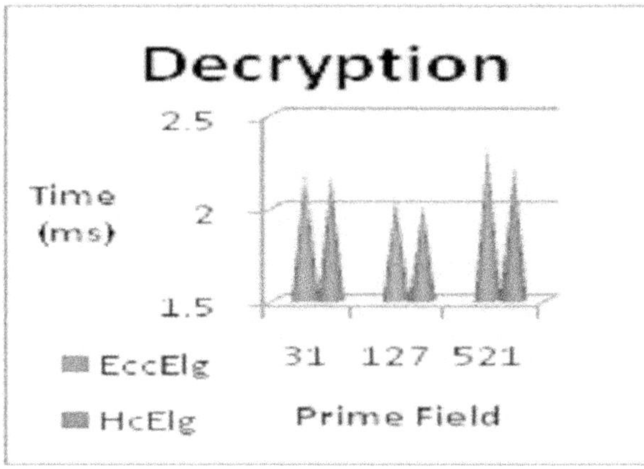

FIGURE 6.8 Decryption time – EccElg and HcElg.

round is process performed by HCDH in which it has public and private keys in every round in alternate way. The procedure of HCDH public key is used to initiate the first round process followed by second round process by private key. Every round of HCAES makes unbreakable cipher text, and finally 10th round process of cipher text is by private key (Figures 6.9 and 6.10). Authentication and key generation algorithms are combined together to produce key for HC(DSADH) to reduce the data size and for faster computation of key generation than genus 1 curve.

In the IoMT, the HC (DSADH) is responsible for verifying the identity of users before generating keys for the group members. This method proves efficiency through various attacks. Related key attack is failed in this cryptosystem, owing to the fact that key generation is derived by HC(DSDH). In medical information encryption phase, HCAES enables the completion of outsourced encryption operations without revealing the content of patient-sensitive information. In this cryptosystem, HC(DSDH AES) security is assured in effective way.

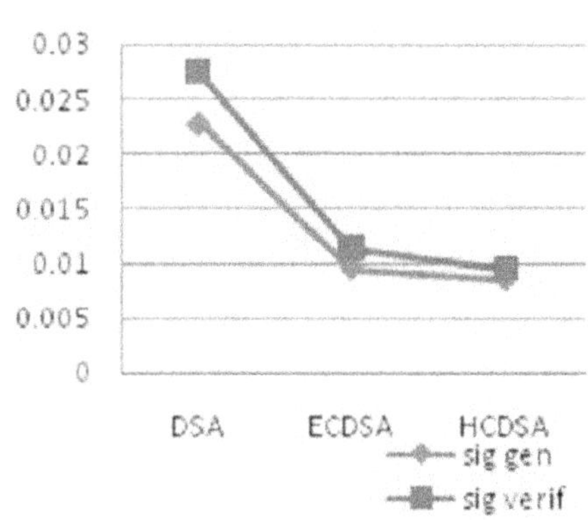

FIGURE 6.9 Digital signature generation and verification through hyperelliptic curve.

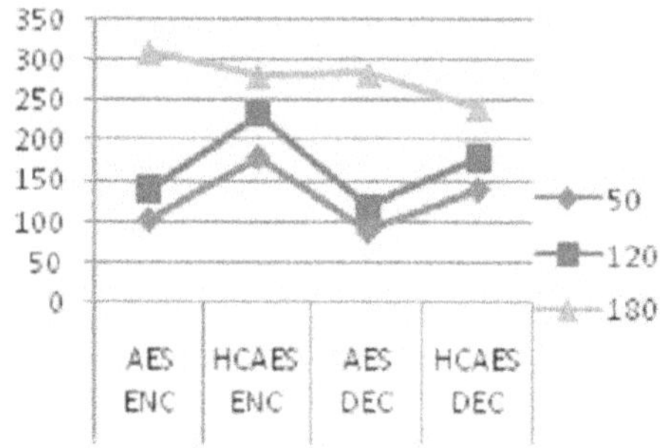

FIGURE 6.10 Symmetric and asymmetric algorithms of AES and DH through hyperelliptic curve (Alphonse and Kavitha, 2019).

The outcome of the recommended approach is evaluated using the genus 2 hyperelliptic curve result that produces the group size 2^{256}, field size 2^{128}, and the security level 2^{128}. It is considered to the advantage of genus 2 curve which is much smaller base field than genus 1 curve in the scalar multiplication. The time taken to execute group member authentication with key generation AES and HCAES were computed. Better execution time is taken for HCDS than the elliptic curve-based DSA and DH. It proves the efficiency of the cryptosystem.

6.2.5 An Efficient Arithmetic on Burnside Curve–Based Cryptography

The Burnside curve is represented over a Finite Field (Fp), a set of points (x, y) as a projective curve with singularity, and the suggested Burnside (B) curve derives new parametrization for elliptic curves. The discriminate of B is $\Delta \neq 0$. Better performance is ensured by an intriguing characteristic of the endomorphism ring with B curve in kummer line–based scalar multiplication via Montgomery ladder algorithm and computation time is minimized by using 2^{127-1} Mersenne prime. Figure 6.9 shows different execution time for DSA,

EcDSA, and HCDSA algorithm (Alphonse, 2021). Figure 6.10 shows different algorithms with different block size execution time.

Niranjanamurthy and Chahar (2013) suggest that rational numbers can serve as an approximate solution to the challenges posed by irrational numbers in scalar multiplication.

The generalization of curves has used genus 2 class numbers 1, 4, and 6; however, genus >1 and class number 2 is never taken into account in cryptosystem. Following examination, a novel curve known as the Burnside curve was discovered. Its properties include class number 2, minimum endomorphism, genus >1, and computing complexity of $6s + 12m$, all of which prove the cryptosystem's efficiency compared to Rangarajan et al. (2013).

The B curve can be represented as

$$B : y^2 = x(x^4 - 1) \tag{6.13}$$

Let L and M represent points on the B curve, where $y = mx + c$. The derivation is used to acquire $x3$, $y3$ from B curve (Alphonse (2021). This point intersects the curve B at point N.

Point Addition Operation

Taking into consideration that the addition operation uses points L and M,
$z = 1$, x_1 *is computed with respect to the projective coordinates.*

$$x_1 = x_1/z_1,\, x_2 = x_2/z_2$$

Let $L\ (x_1,\ y_1)$, $M\ (x_2,\ y_2) \in GF\ (p)$, where $x_1 \neq x_{2,}$ then compute $N = L + M$

$$x_3 = (c^2/(x_1 x_2)) + (((x_1 * x_2)/3) * (x^2 + x^2 + x_1 * x_2)) + (2(x_1 + x_2)^3/27) \quad (6.14)$$

$$y_3 = s(x_3 - x_1) + y_1 \quad (6.15)$$

where $s = (y_2 - y_1)/(x_2 - x_1)$

Point Doubling Operation

Let $L(x_1,\ y_1) \in GF\ (p)$, where $L \neq -L$, $2L = (x_3,\ y_3)$

$$x_3 = (c^2/x^2) + x^4 + 16x^3/27) \quad (6.16)$$

$$y_3 = s(x_3 - x_1) + y_1 \quad (6.17)$$

where $s = 5x^4 - 1/2y$. Let L represent the point on the curve; the addition is the definition

of the multiplication operation at point L.

$k * L = L + L + L + \cdots + L$, which means L is added k number of times.

The B curve demonstrates a superior performance stability, offering high security with low computational cost and time. The performance analysis of the B curve and ECC with different prime field was carried out, with implementation of DH and ElGamal schemes.

The noteworthy bit of the secure key is exposed from the accepted fault when $q * k = (x3,\ y3)$, which is calculated using the exceptional points of L and M, but it is unable to yield the right value,. This indicates a scalar multiplication error when order N is small, a subgroup attack focusing on the points on the curve has been utilized to attain data. There won't be a successful subgroup assault if the prime order on the curve is massive. Therefore, the subgroup attack is impotent to extract the secret key in the proposed B curve because it has points and a large prime order. Burnside curve–based RSA increases system efficiency and achieves high levels of security; nevertheless, it must be developed by reducing public key cryptosystem key sizes, as noted by Bos et al. (2009) and Huang and Wang (2015).

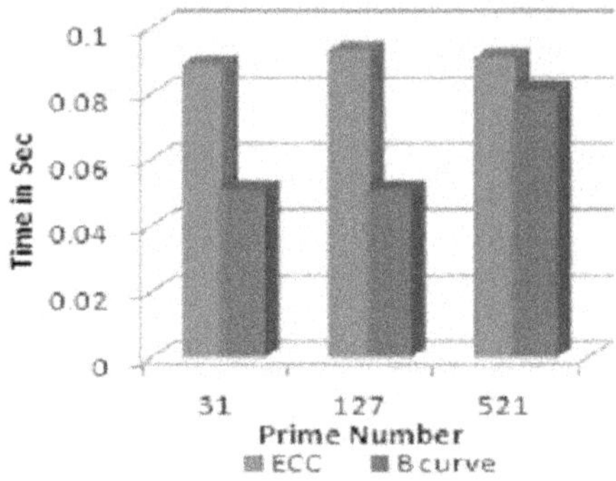

FIGURE 6.11 Encryption time – ECC and B curve.

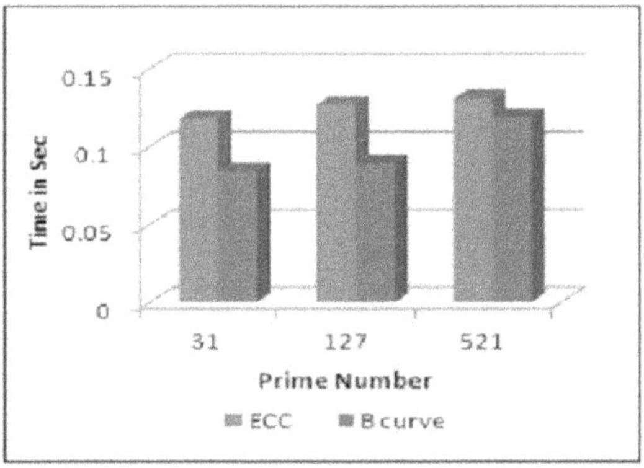

FIGURE 6.12 Decryption time – ECC and B curve.

The degree of security is determined by the curve's derivation points as well as the hardness of the discrete logarithmic problem (DLP) on group over Burnside curve. Burnside curve cryptography implementation yields smaller key sizes than conventional RSA, with 61, 107, 127, and 159 bit employed as Mersenne primes (Niranjanamurthy and Chahar, 2013; Singh et al., 2013). Figures 6.11 and 6.12 show that ECC and B curve key generation and overall performance of the algorithms RSA key and *B* curve key sizes are shown in Figures 6.13 and 6.14 (Alphonse et al., 2021).

The RSA key size rises when a little quantity of prime increases, but the *B* curve key size remains parallel to the prime number raised. The graph shows that the 120 key size of B curve cryptography is equivalent to the 1,024 bit RSA key.

6.3 CONCLUSION

The study has identified IoMT security systems, and effective solutions have been suggested. Sensitive medical data stored in IoMT needs to be securely transferred

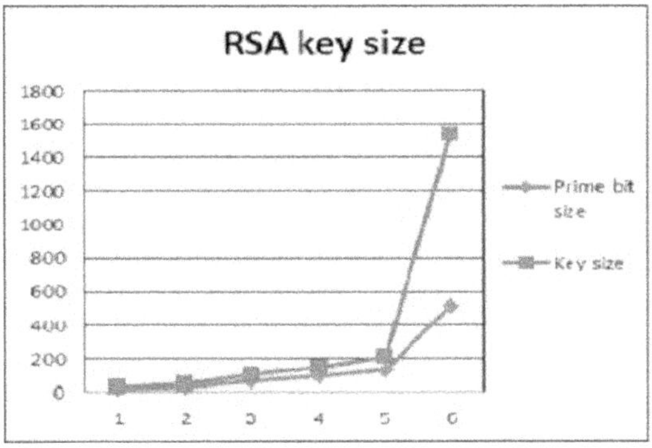

FIGURE 6.13 Different key size by RSA.

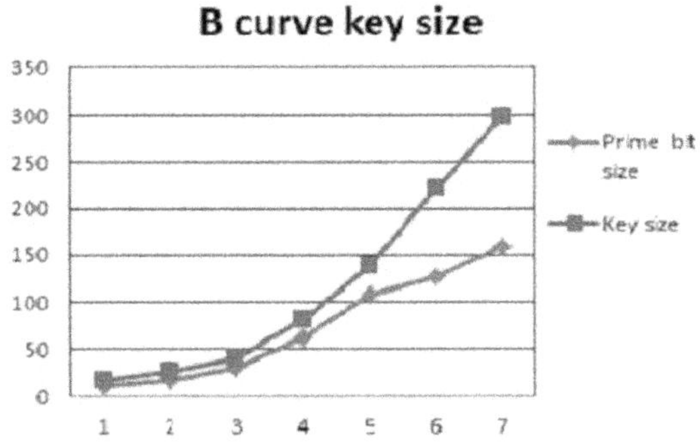

FIGURE 6.14 Different key size by B curve.

and accessed quickly. The hybrid algorithm (AES DH)HC, which combines AES HC and DH HC, is responsible for achieving it. Decentralized group key agreement with HC-based DH algorithm is denoted by (*DSGK HCDH*). This method repairs the security flaws during generation and distribution of group key. The strength of the method is proved through user anonymity, data confidentiality, and backward/forward security. Scalable group key approach is far more secure than other levels of security when used with HcDSA and HcElg algorithms. A comprehensive review of suggested validation scheme's security and prescribed analysis have demonstrated its effectiveness against known potential threats, hash function attacks, per-message secret attacks, and solution of the HcDLP problem. Subgroup attack is unable to obtain information by using a Burnside curve cryptography system based on a kummer surface. Because of its low power needs and smaller key length, the RSA cryptosystem on the B curve is well suited for Internet of Medical Things applications, offering significantly improved security performance.

REFERENCES

Adedeji, K. B., & Famoriji, J. O. (2014). Investigating the effects of varying the key size on the performance of AES algorithm for encryption of data over a communication channel. *International Journal of Applied Information Systems*, *7*(8), 6–10.

Alphonse, P. J. A. (2021). Security enhancement through efficient arithmetic on novel curve based cryptography. *Turkish Online Journal of Qualitative Inquiry*, *12*(5), 2529.

Alphonse, P. J. A., & Reddy, Y. V. (2019). A method for obtaining authenticated scalable and efficient group key agreement for wireless ad-hoc networks. *Cluster Computing*, *22*(Suppl 2), 3145–3151. *Cluster Computing*, 1–7.

Alphonse, P. J. A., Pulagara, P. S. B., & Kavitha, S. (2021). Enhanced e-commerce security using RSA through Burnside curve cryptography. *Turkish Online journal of Qualitative Inquiry, 12*(5), 2537–2548.

Bernstein, D. J., & Lange, T. (2014). Hyper-and-elliptic-curve cryptography. *LMS Journal of Computation and Mathematics*, *17*(A), 181–202.

Bernstein, D. J., Birkner, P., Joye, M., Lange, T., & Peters, C. (2008). *Twisted Edwards curves*. Progress in Cryptology–AFRICACRYPT 2008: First International Conference on Cryptology in Africa, Casablanca, Morocco, June 11–14, 2008. Proceedings 1. Springer Berlin Heidelberg, pp. 389–405.

Bos, J., Kaihara, M., Kleinjung, T., Lenstra, A. K., & Montgomery, P. L. (2009). *On the security of 1024-bit RSA and 160-bit elliptic curve cryptography*. Technical Report.

Huang, X., & Wang, W. (2015). A novel and efficient design for an RSA cryptosystem with a very large key size. *IEEE Transactions on Circuits and Systems II: Express Briefs*, *62*(10), 972–976.

Jaiswal, P., & Tripathi, S. (2017). An authenticated group key transfer protocol using elliptic curve cryptography. *Peer-to-Peer Networking and Applications*, *10*(4), 857–864.

Kavitha, S., & Alphonse, P. J. A. (2019). A hybrid cryptosystem to enhance security in IoT health care system. *International Journal of Wireless and Microwave Technologies*, *11*(1), 1–10.

Kavitha, S., Alphonse, P. J. A., & Reddy, Y. V. (2019). An improved authentication and security on efficient generalized group key agreement using hyper elliptic curve based public key cryptography for IoT health care system. *Journal of Medical Systems*, *43*(8), 260.

Mathur A, Newe T, Elgenaidi W, Rao M, Dooly G, Toal D.(2017). A secure end-to-end IoT solution. Sensors and Actuators A: Physical. Aug 15;263:291-9.

Menezes, A., van Oorschot, P., & Vanstone, S. (1996). *Handbook of applied cryptography*. Jaypee Medical.

Niranjanamurthy, M., & Chahar, D. (2013). The study of e-commerce security issues and solutions. *International Journal of Advanced Research in Computer and Communication Engineering*, *2*(7), 2885–2895.

Rangarajan, S., Ram, N. S., & Krishna, N. V. (2013). Securing SMS using cryptography. *International Journal of Computer Science and Information Technologies (IJCSIT)*, *4*(2), 285–288.

Singh, S., Garg, A., & Sachdeva, A. (2013). Comparison of cryptographic algorithms: ECC and RSA. *International Journal of Computer Science and Communication Engineering*, *2*(1), 211–216.

Stallings, W. (2017). *Cryptography and network security: Principles and practice* (7th ed.). Pearson.

Thangavelu, S., & Vijaykumar, V. (2016). Efficient modified Elliptic Curve Diffie-Hellman algorithm for VoIP networks. *International Arab Journal of Information Technology (IAJIT)*, *13*(5), 559–566.

Veltri, L., Cirani, S., Busanelli, S., & Ferrari, G. (2013). A novel batch-based group key management protocol applied to the internet of things. *Ad Hoc Networks*, *11*(8), 2724–2737.
Xin, M. (2015). *A mixed encryption algorithm used in internet of things security trans- mission system*. 2015 International Conference on Cyber-Enabled Distributed Computing and Knowledge Discovery. IEEE, pp. 62–65.

7 Post-Processing of Unmanned Aerial Vehicle Images of Search and Rescue Mission

Vaideghy A., Thiyagarajan C., and Sudha R.

7.1 INTRODUCTION

Natural disasters (e.g., droughts, earthquakes, floods, storms, landslides) are catastrophic phenomena with atmospheric, geological, and hydrological sources that can result in fatalities, property destruction, and social and environmental disorder. One such natural calamity is intense shaking of earth's surfaces, which lead to earthquakes. Earthquakes occur when the earth's surface experiences a sudden release of stress. The tectonic plates exist beneath the earth's surface slide one over the other, causing the ground surface to shake. Structure damage, short circuits, bridge and highway failure, and a major release of combustible compounds via gas lines and factories all are consequences of earthquakes.

The response measures of earthquake include alerting the emergency services like medical facilities, ambulance, police, and fire department for immediate help. Search, rescue and evacuation processes need to be carried out immediately after a disaster strikes a certain area or building. These are the most immediate critical operations that are usually performed by the local volunteers, voluntary organizations, and the emergency agencies which consume time.

Most of the post-disaster rescue measures are now done with computer vision using drones. *Computer vision* is the capacity of computers to perceive images and videos on their own. It is a field that studies how computers can perceive digital images or videos at a high level. From an engineering standpoint, it aims at understanding and automating operations that the human visual system is capable of. It involves acquiring, processing, analyzing, and understanding visual data to extract meaningful information, which can then be used to make decisions or take actions. Computer vision aids in increasing the accuracy and decreasing the response times in search and rescue missions. Almost all unmanned aerial vehicle (UAV) images used by disaster management committee are captured during adverse weather conditions

 DOI: 10.1201/9781003476344-7

which are with either high or low humidity, fog, haze, and lighting effect that affects the clarity or resolution. This eventually provides a blurry image.

This chapter proposes a method based on contrast-limited adaptive histogram equalization (CLAHE) and deblurring using Gaussian blur kernel to remove the noises from the obtained images and improve their quality.

7.1.1 Objectives of the Work

The information acquired by the rescue team from UAV-captured images are altered by environmental noises such as atmospheric condition and high wind, which ultimately result in quality degradation. In order to overcome the blurriness and improve the quality of these images, deblurring of UAV-captured images is necessary so that the processed images could help the rescue team to save the victims during any kind of natural calamities in less time. Additionally, to restore the images captured from UAV, to deblur the images affected by noise, to use the processed image in search and rescue mission process, and to use object detection technique in order to analyze the results, the proposed work is recommended.

7.1.2 Proposed Work

Aerial imagery of drones can play an important role when large area is to be covered, when limited resources are available, or in critical weather conditions in search and rescue operations. But the images captured by the drones may be affected by weather conditions (fog, haze) and motion, which slows the rescuing process during disaster. Two main problems identified with aerial imagery is that the images might be blurred or fogged. Thus, the images need processing which helps the Rescue Committee obtain clear results and faster rescuing in less time.

7.2 LITERATURE SURVEY

Persson and Andersson [1] investigated whether an UAV equipped with positional sensors and a high-resolution camera can be used to take aerial photographs and create coherent orthophotos in real time or near real time using mobile devices. Three different seam stitching algorithms are tested and compared in terms of speed, accuracy, and visual appearance. The entire mission is carried out without the involvement of any humans. However, the outcomes of those three methods are unsatisfactory. Cropping is their first method which ignored any color or rotational differences in the photos. If the photos have significant rotational differences, the seam will be visible. Their second method is pixel matching. The pixel match method provides the best visual solution, but it is much more difficult to implement. In pixel matching, all photos at once require too many resources, hence the iPad run out of memory and the app gets crashed. However, in some images, the algorithm was unable to find matching features, resulting in stitching failure and no real-world results. Using OpenCV for pixel matching full-scale aerial photograph is also not ideal.

Saravanan [2] converts a color image to a grayscale image using a proposed algorithm that uses luminance to approximate RGB values. RGB components are approximated by three values: lightness, chroma, and hue, added with chrominance value, and average of these four values resulted in perceptually and structurally good grayscale image quality. This algorithm is useful in a variety of applications where a high-quality grayscale image is required.

Yadav [3] presents a novel algorithm for real-time video surveillance systems that is based on the contrast-adaptive histogram equalization enhancement technique. The images are fused into a new frame, and the histogram equalization method is used to adjust intensity values separately for the background and foreground images.

Priyanka et al. [4] propose a deblurring image restoration technique using a Gaussian filter. A Gaussian filter is used to blur the images first and remove noise. The smoothing gradation is determined by the quality eccentricity of the Gaussian. To obtain a blurred image, various reasonable noise is added, and the deblurring method is used. When this image filtering is enforced, it removes the additional noise as well.

Azouaoui et al. [5] propose a multi-object detection system based on detectors in cascade and HOG. The detection system was tested offline on well-known datasets as well as online on a car-like mobile robot navigating a real road. The obtained results show a detection rate of 74 and an average precision of 0.639.

Mbaitiga et al. [6] describe how to detect human bodies quickly at a disaster site using image processing from an UAV. The RGB color space was converted to HSV, and the morphological method's opening and closing operations were carried out. The experiments were carried out both indoors and outdoors.

Sarosa et al. [7] used the YOLO algorithm for the detection of victims of natural disasters. The dataset consisted of 200 images, 100 for training and 100 for testing. Training data were collected up to the epoch of 3,000. However, several factors influence the detection results, including the background of the object in the image, the position of the object, and the clarity of the image.

All the works have limitations either with output clarity or with the system requirements. The techniques used so far for image processing are inferred and a comparative study is done to find the methods with best performance measures.

7.3 SCOPE OF THE WORK

The aim of this work is to overcome the difficulties faced in the traditional methods of deblurring. The proposed method uses CLAHE for image enhancement and Gaussian blur for deblurring which shows better results by improving the quality. The accuracy is then analyzed by detecting the disaster victims.

7.4 LIMITATIONS

The dataset for training the system is constrained due to only the recent use of UAV photos for search and rescue missions in disaster response. To broaden the use of this work in the future, we will need a large dataset to obtain a high level of accuracy.

7.5 EXISTING WORK

The use of drones has swiftly evolved over the last decade, with applications ranging from agriculture to commerce to disaster management and humanitarian aid. Unfortunately, there is still a lack of proof of its use in major disasters. In 2013, India's NDMA employed drones for the first time in disaster management. Drone application in disasters are classified into four categories: (1) mapping, (2) search and rescue, (3) transportation, and (4) training.

Time is a vital aspect in the success of first responders in disaster situations or search and rescue scenarios. Unmanned systems have the possibility to provide new capabilities for these scenarios decreasing the response time. Due to their flexible deployment possibilities and capabilities, UAVs are ideal candidates for novel localization systems when victims are sparsely distributed in large and/or difficult-to-reach areas. One problem with these scenarios is that the disaster may have changed the environment which has an impact on victim identification and crew reaction time.

7.6 RESEARCH METHODOLOGY

The major goal of this project is to use deblurring technique to reconstruct the UAV photos that were captured. The processed image is then utilized as information by rescuers. Due to erratic environments or the lack of coordinated actions by various agencies, accurate data collection may be extremely difficult during a disaster. The use of drones in a disaster has the following benefits: they reduce the time required to locate victims as well as the time required for searching a large area, in addition to providing critical information to rescuers. Drones are critical tools for acquiring aerial images. Aerial photographs are extremely valuable in planning relief and rescue activities since they provide quick and accurate information about the disaster-stricken area. However, the image taken is prone to quality degradation in severe weather conditions or distorted landscapes, and is rarely configured with solid camera platforms. This creates a problem when gathering on-site information. In broader terms, aerial image processing is necessary to collect coherent information about the ground surface.

The suggested method improves image quality by using CLAHE for image enhancement and Gaussian blur for deblurring. The accuracy is then assessed by identifying disaster victims.

7.6.1 Computer Vision

Computer vision is the capacity of computers to perceive images and videos on their own. It is a field that studies how computers can perceive digital images or videos at a high level. From an engineering standpoint, it aims at understanding and automating operations that the human visual system is capable of. Computer vision tasks include methods for acquiring, processing, analyzing, and understanding digital images, and extraction of high-dimensional data from the real world in order to produce numerical or symbolic information.

Image restoration is a common computer vision task which refers to the restoration or reconstruction of faded images that have been captured or stored in an improper manner, leading to a loss of quality of the image. Typical image restoration processes involve the reduction of additive noise via mathematical tools, while at times, reconstruction requires major changes, leading to further analysis and the use of image inpainting. In image inpainting, damaged parts of an image are filled with the help of generative models that make an estimate of what the image is trying to convey. Often, the restoration process is followed by a colorization process that colors the subject of the picture (if black and white) in the most realistic manner possible.

7.6.2 Edge Enhancement Filter

Edge enhancement is an image processing filter that enhances the edge contrast of an image to improve its apparent sharpness. This feature has the effect of creating subtle bright and dark highlights on either side of any edges in the image, leading the edge to look more defined. Edge enhancement filters enhance the local discontinuities at the boundaries of different objects (edges) in the image. An edge in a signal is normally defined as the transition in the intensity or amplitude of that signal. Unlike some forms of image sharpening, edge enhancement does not enhance subtle detail which may appear in more uniform areas of the image, such as texture or grain which appears in flat or smooth areas of the image. The benefit of this is that imperfections in the image reproduction, such as grain or noise, or imperfections in the subject, such as natural imperfections on a person's skin, are not made more obvious by the process. A drawback to this is that the image may begin to look less natural, because the apparent sharpness of the overall image has increased but the level of detail in flat, smooth areas has not.

As with other forms of image sharpening, edge enhancement is only capable of improving the perceived sharpness or acutance of an image. The enhancement is not completely reversible, and as such some detail in the image is lost as a result of filtering. Further sharpening operations on the resulting image compound the loss of detail, leading to artifacts such as ringing. An example of this can be seen when an image that has already had edge enhancement applied, such as the picture on a DVD video, has further edge enhancement applied by the DVD player it is played on, and possibly also by the television it is displayed on. Essentially, the first edge enhancement filter creates new edges on either side of the existing edges, which are then further enhanced.

7.6.3 CLAHE

Adaptive histogram equalization (AHE) is a computer image processing technique used to improve contrast in images. It differs from ordinary histogram equalization in that the adaptive method computes several histograms, each corresponding to a

- Kernel for `ImageFilter.EDGE_ENHANCE:`

```
(
    -1, -1, -1,
    -1, 10, -1,
    -1, -1, -1
)
```

FIGURE 7.1 AHE representation.

distinct section of the image, and uses them to redistribute the lightness values of the image. It is therefore suitable for improving the local contrast and enhancing the definitions of edges in each region of an image. But AHE over amplifies noise in relatively homogeneous regions of an image. Figure 7.1 describes the AHE representation. CLAHE is a variant of adaptive histogram equalization in which the contrast amplification is limited, so as to reduce this problem of noise amplification.

7.6.4 Median Filter

A median filter is a non-linear filter in which each output sample is computed as the median value of the input samples under the window—that is, the result is the middle value after the input values have been sorted. Ordinarily, an odd number of taps is used. The median filter is a non-linear digital filtering technique, often used to remove noise from an image or a signal. Such noise reduction is a typical pre-processing step to improve the results of later processing (for example, edge detection

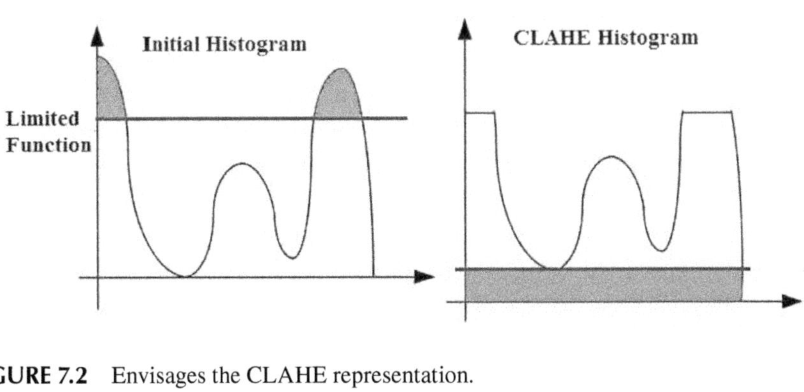

FIGURE 7.2 Envisages the CLAHE representation.

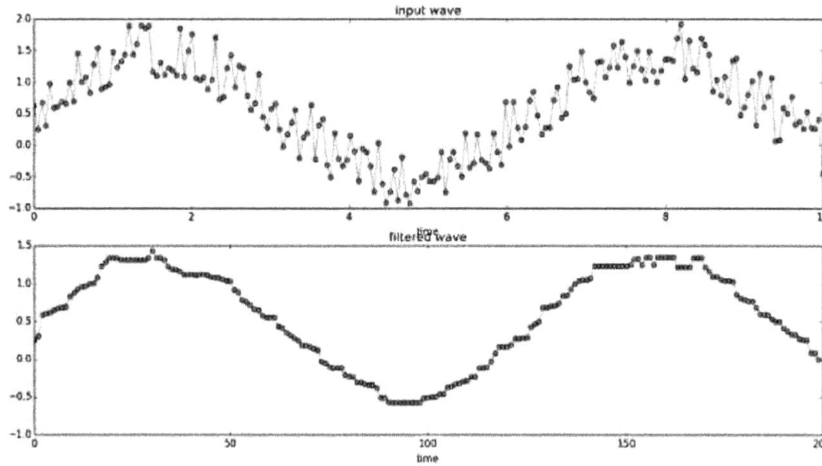

FIGURE 7.3 Pixel value is replaced by the median value of the neighboring pixel.

on an image). It is also known as non-linear filtering. It is used to eliminate salt and pepper noise. Here the pixel value is replaced by the median value of the neighboring pixel. The same is represented in Figure 7.3.

7.6.5 Gaussian Deblurring

Blurring is a commonly used visual effect in image processing. One of the most common blurs used in this field is the Gaussian blur in which each pixel in the image we wish to blur is considered independently, and its value change depending on its own value, and those of its surroundings, based on a filter matrix called a kernel.

The kernel consists of a rectangular array of numbers that follow a Gaussian distribution, also known as a normal distribution, or a bell curve. The rectangular kernel consists of values that are higher in the middle and drop off toward the outer edges of the square array, like the height of a bell curve in two dimensions. The kernel corresponds to the number of pixels we consider when blurring each individual pixel. Blur increases, as the kernel size increases.

7.6.6 YOLO

YOLO is a state-of-the-art, real-time object detection system. In YOLO, an input picture is distributed to a system of S × S grids. The detection of the object depends on every grid of the input image. Grid cells are employed to predict targets inside boundary boxes. Five parameters are predicted for every boundary box. These five elements are i, j, k, l, and c. In the input picture, the center of target inside the box is denoted by i and j coordinates. Here, k, l, and c represent height, width, and score for confidence, respectively. c is measured as the probability of containing the target inside boundary box. For every cell in the network, it computes confidence for n

bounding boxes. YOLO v1 has many limitations. Therefore, the use of YOLO v1 is restricted to some extent. Limitations of YOLO version1 are based on the closeness of the objects in the picture. If the objects appear as a cluster, they cannot find the small objects. Yolo v2 uses darknet19, which has convolutional layers in it. Since there are many limitations in Yolo v1 and Yolo v2, Yolo v3 has been used for detection in our system which results in better efficiency and accuracy and also needs in less processing time.

7.6.6.1 YOLOv3

One of the advanced variants of YOLO is version 3 that uses logistic regression to compute the target score. It gives the score for all targets in each boundary box. YOLO v3 can give the multilabel classification because it uses a logistic classifier for each class in place of the soft-max layer used in YOLO v2. YOLO v3 uses darknet 53. It has 53 layers of convolution. These layers are more in depth compared to darknet 19 used in YOLO v2. Darknet-53 contains mainly 3×3 and 1×1 filters.

7.7 SYSTEM IMPLEMENTATION

The proposed system uses computer vision for image processing. CLAHE is used for image enhancement and deblurring is done with the help of Gaussian blur. The result is then checked for accuracy using human detection. YOLOv3 is used for human detection.

The UAVs and aerial images have been used over the past decade for search and rescue operations. But the images captured may be affected due to critical weather conditions and erratic environments. Hence, processing of UAV images is a great advantage which decreases response time and provides accurate information to the rescuers about the disaster-stricken area. The solution is divided into three phases. In the first phase, image is restored and enhanced. Figure 7.4 depicts the system architecture of YOLOv3.

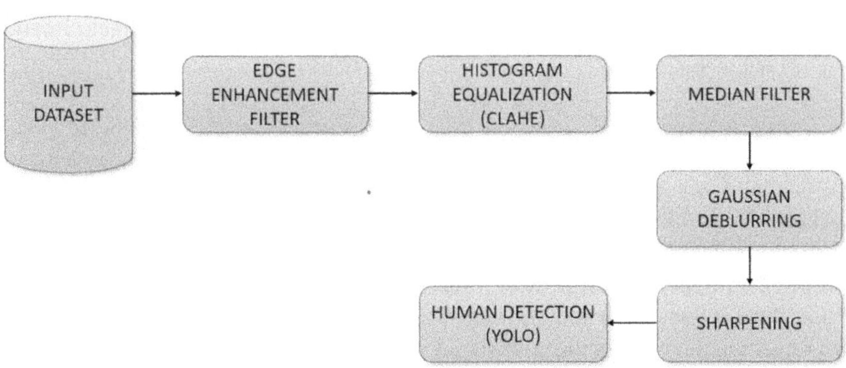

FIGURE 7.4 System architecture of YOLOv3.

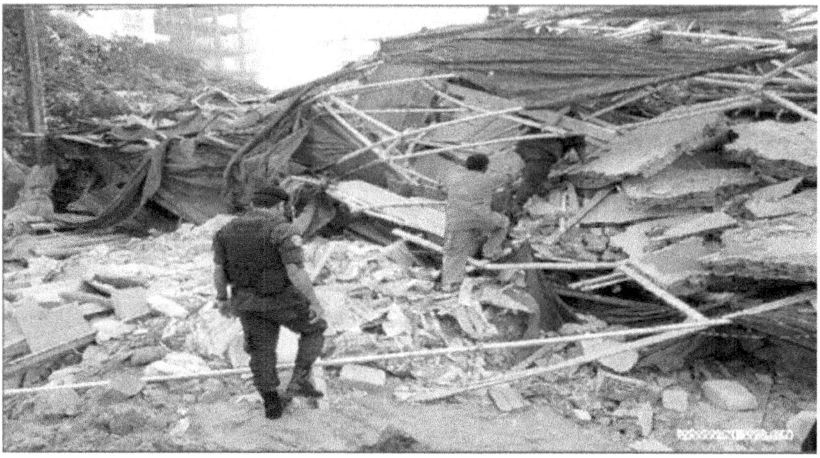

FIGURE 7.5 Sample input image.

7.7.1 Dataset

The dataset comes from a public accessible repository—Kaggle. Data images were gathered consisting of UAV images captured during disasters. Here earthquake and flood datasets are taken into account. Sample input image is highlighted in Figure 7.5.

7.7.2 Image Enhancement

The input image is divided into small blocks called "tiles" (tile size is 8 × 8 by default in OpenCV). Then for each of these blocks are histograms equalized as usual. So, in a small area, histogram would confine to a small region (unless there is noise). If noise is there, it will be amplified. To avoid this, contrast limiting is applied. If any histogram bin is above the specified contrast limit (by default 40 in OpenCV), those pixels are clipped and distributed uniformly to other bins before applying histogram equalization. After equalization, to remove artifacts in tile borders, bilinear interpolation is applied. Application is represented in Figure 7.6.

7.7.3 Median Filter

The median filter considers each pixel in the image in turn and looks at its nearby neighbors to decide whether or not it is representative of its surroundings. Instead of simply replacing the pixel value with the mean of neighboring pixel values, it replaces it with the median of those values. The median is calculated by first sorting all the pixel values from the surrounding neighborhood into numerical order and then replacing the pixel being considered with the middle pixel value. Application is represented in Figure 7.7.

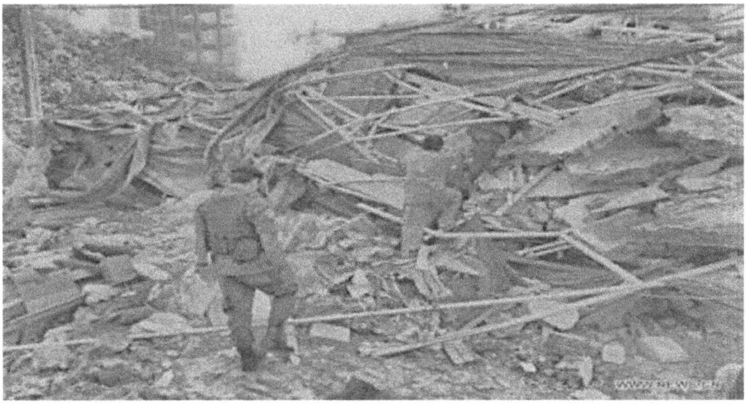

FIGURE 7.6 Enhanced image of input image.

7.7.4 Image Deblurring

The Gaussian blur compared to other filters uses unique kernel which provides less weight to distant pixels. When we convolve a matrix with another matrix, the matrices should be of the same dimensions. This means that we cannot apply a 2D convolution to our 3D (because of the color channels) matrix. Gaussian blur convolution is applied iteratively to the image. Then the image is sharpened and the function returns an image that is noticeably sharper with none of the color distortions. Figure 7.8 is the deblurred image of input image.

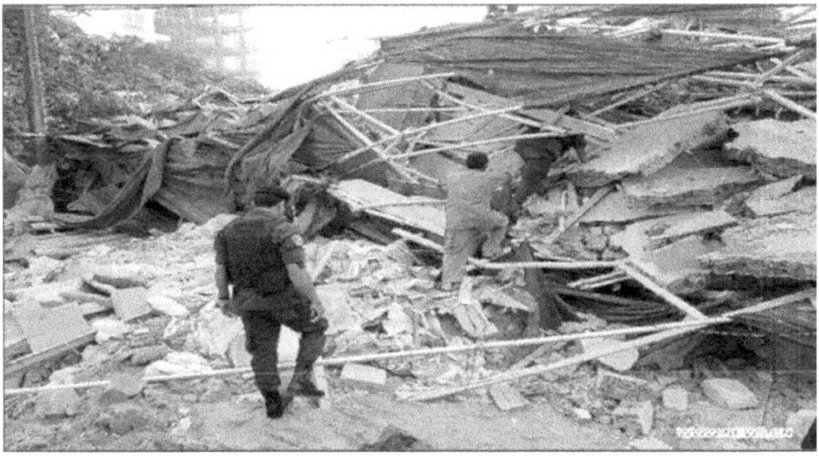

FIGURE 7.7 Median filter output of input image.

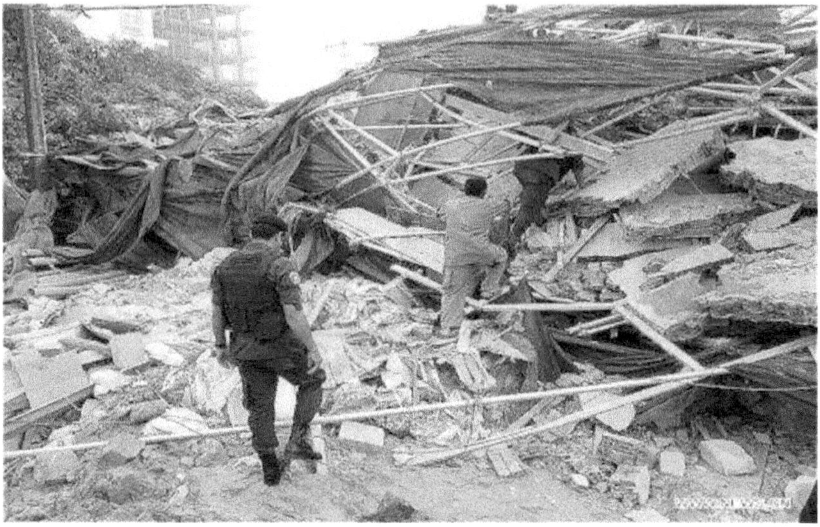

FIGURE 7.8 Deblurred image of input image.

7.8 HUMAN DETECTION

Initially weights, cfg and coco.names files are downloaded. Confidence threshold and non-max suppression threshold are set. OpenCV darknet module reads the model configuration file and weights file which find the objects in the image and assigns bounding boxes. The bounding boxes are compared with the threshold values and the object is detected. Object detection is a computer technology related to computer vision and image processing that deals with detecting instances of semantic objects of a certain class (such as humans, buildings, or cars) in digital images and videos [1]. Well-researched domains of object detection include face detection and pedestrian detection. Object detection has applications in many areas of computer vision, including image retrieval and video surveillance.

Every object class has its own special features that help in classifying the class—for example, all circles are round. Object class detection uses these special features. For example, when looking for circles, objects that are at a particular distance from a point (i.e., the center) are sought. Similarly, when looking for squares, objects that are perpendicular at corners and have equal side lengths are needed. A similar approach is used for face identification where eyes, nose, and lips can be found and features like skin color and distance between eyes can be found.

7.9 RESULT AND DISCUSSION

The images captured by the drones may be affected by weather conditions (fog, haze) and motion, which slows the rescuing process during disaster. Thus, the images need processing which helps the Rescue Committee to get clear results and faster rescuing in less time. From the proposed system, it is inferred that the accuracy of human detection in deblurred image is higher than that of original, unprocessed image and has detected persons who were not detected in original image.

7.10. CONCLUSION AND FUTURE ENHANCEMENT

The aim of this work is to process the UAV images which can be used for search and rescue missions during disaster. The efficiency and accuracy of the proposed method is verified by detecting humans in the images. The accuracy of human detection is higher in the output image. The system can be scaled to detect humans using facial recognition and other body parts. The system can also be improvised by including human counting which can be used as information by the Rescue Committee to send help accordingly. This system can be improved further to be used with video datasets.

REFERENCES

1. Persson, D., and J. Andersson. 2016. "Real-Time Image Processing on Handheld Devices and UAV." Dissertation.
2. Chandran, Saravanan. 2010. "Color Image to Grayscale Age Conversion." In *Proceedings of the 2010 2nd International Conference on Computer Engineering and Applications*, 196–199. https://doi.org/10.1109/ICCEA.2010.192.
3. Yadav, Garima. 2014. "Contrast Limited Adaptive Histogram Equalization Based Enhancement for Real-Time Video System." In *2014 International Conference on Advances in Computing, Communications and Informatics (ICACCI)*. https://doi.org/10.1109/ICACCI.2014.6968381.
4. Priyanka, Rishabh Shukla, and Laxmi Shrivastava. 2020. "Image Restoration of Image with Gaussian Filter." *International Research Journal of Engineering and Technology (IRJET)* 7 (12): Article V7I1299.
5. Azouaoui, O., A. Chayeb, Noureddine Ouadah, Z. Tobal, and Mustapha Lakrouf. 2014. "HOG-Based Multi-Object Detection for Urban Navigation." In *2014 IEEE 17th International Conference on Intelligent Transportation Systems (ITSC)*. https://doi.org/10.1109/ITSC.2014.6958165.
6. Mbaitiga, Zacharie, Satoshi Fujii, and Minori Shimoji. 2017. "Rapid Human Body Detection in Disaster Sites Using Image Processing from Unmanned Aerial Vehicle (UAV) Cameras." *International Journal of Robotics and Automation* 3: 96–101.
7. Sarosa, Moechammad, Nipuna Muna, and Rohadi Erfan. 2021. "Detection of Natural Disaster Victims Using You Only Look Once (YOLO)." *IOP Conference Series: Materials Science and Engineering* 1098 (3): 032076. https://doi.org/10.1088/1757-899X/1098/3/032076.

8 Revolutionizing Mental Health Care

The Transformative Power of Internet of Medical Things (IoMT): A Comprehensive Overview and Case Studies

Abilash K., Sindhuja Manisha Kamini P., Ruchi Joshi, and Ayisha Nejili

8.1 INTRODUCTION TO IOMT IN MENTAL HEALTH CARE

The phrase "Internet of Medical Things" (IoMT) refers to online networks that link medical applications and devices to healthcare IT systems. The foundation of IoMT, machine-to-machine communication, is made possible by medical equipment that include Wi-Fi. Furthermore, IoMT devices connect to cloud services like Amazon Web Services so that recorded data may be saved and examined there. Healthcare IoT is another name for IoMT (Gao et al., 2020). IoMT in mental health care has transformed the way medical professionals diagnose, treat, and follow up patients. By using IoMT technologies, mental health care providers can access real-time data that will lead to more accurate assessments and personalized interventions. Continuous monitoring of the health status of an unexpectedly large number of patients during the pre-and post-infection stages is extremely important. Since the COVID-19 pandemic, both patients and caregivers have effectively acclimated to remote patient monitoring, screening, and treatment via telehealth facilitated by IoMT. The IoMT-based smart gadgets are becoming more and more commonplace, especially in light of the current worldwide pandemic (Joyce et al., 2023). However, given the enormous amount of demand, the healthcare industry is anticipated to be one of the most difficult industries for IoMT. A collection of biomedical devices and applications that are able to interface with healthcare data management infrastructures is known as the Internet of Medical Things (Patle, 2024). By strengthening the bond between patients and their doctors and enabling the sharing of medical information over a secure platform, it may decrease needless hospital visits and ease the burden on

DOI: 10.1201/9781003476344-8

medical practices. IoMT and wearable technology are also the foundation of telemedicine, which has attracted a lot of interest in recent years and remotely monitors patients from their homes. With this type of care, patients can avoid having to visit a hospital or a doctor's clinic every time they have a medical query or experience a change in their health. From a commercial perspective, the rising cost of medical services might be a major obstacle. Additionally, the aging of the global population in many parts of the world is contributing to an increase in the prevalence of chronic illnesses (Mathkor et al., 2024). In fact, the likelihood of the current community being more prone to chronic illnesses is greater. It follows that for most individuals, access to healthcare will eventually become costly. Virtual patient care is now feasible, thanks to the Internet of Medical Things, which has also improved biopharmaceutical and healthcare processes. Technologies that concentrate on healthcare sanitation, in particular, help to maintain people's health. Hospitals can speed urgent care and control refrigerator temperatures with the use of IoMT solutions. People use gadgets like heartbeat monitors, pressure sensors, and glucometers, to name but a few, that transmit data to their physicians even when they are not in hospitals. The potential advantages of the IoMT have just lately begun to be assessed, despite the fact that such technical advancements have the potential to be revolutionary. As a matter of fact, Fortune Business Insights projected that the need for IoMT in healthcare would increase dramatically over the following eight years, from $87.62 billion in 2022 to $852.88 billion in 2030.

The length of wait times in emergency rooms has significantly decreased as a result of IoMT advancements. Using object recognition, sonar cameras, and RFID tags, hospital bed occupancy is tracked in real time. This expedites the transfer of patients from an ER to an inpatient facility. This information may be useful to emergency medication technicians (EMTs) who transport patients to hospitals. EMTs can transfer patients to the next hospital that has capacity if there is a space issue at one facility. Detection systems are useful for tracking the many sorts of blood samples that are accessible or the hospital's bloodstream. They also help with inpatient admissions.

This information also aids EMTs in selecting the best hospital for a patient. As soon as a patient enrolls and enters an emergency department, they are given ID wristbands that are activated by IoMT, which track them during their whole stay. Hospitals look at how long patients spend at each stage of the process to find areas for improvement (Gates, 2024). In the future, urgent care services may employ advanced technology in the form of an IoMT-enabled credential that monitors cardiac output, heartbeat, pulse rate, and breathing rate. The gadget notifies clinical practitioners if a patient's temperature unexpectedly increases while they are waiting for an appointment.

Although in the past such circumstances looked hopeless, patients are now being saved from such issues by cutting-edge developments, such as the development of IoMT apps. Technology may make healthcare more easily accessible and reasonably priced, but it is evident that it cannot reverse the effects of aging or lessen the effects of chronic illnesses. Thanks to technology improvements, medical treatment may now mostly take place in the patient's bedroom. The future of IoMT may not be clear to many healthcare businesses. In this chapter, we attempt to cover the need of all people.

8.2 THE ROLE OF IOMT IN DIAGNOSIS AND TREATMENT

IoMT plays a crucial role in improving the accuracy and efficiency of diagnosis in mental health care. Through the use of algorithms and computed data analysis, IoMT can predict minor and major health issues, enabling early intervention and treatment planning. IoMT involves recording medicine orders, hospital admission locations, wearable medical devices that patients can use to communicate with caregivers, and remote patient monitoring for those with long-term or chronic illnesses. Furthermore, medical devices that can be converted to or implemented as IoMT technology include infusion pumps that interface with analytics dashboards and hospital beds equipped with sensors that track patients' vital signs. In pharmacogenomics, fast delivery of individualized treatment plans and current diagnoses are crucial. Using data from the past and present, artificial intelligence (AI) provides real-time solutions by identifying novel approaches to addressing specific conditions. The application of AI-based technologies has the potential to change many aspects of the healthcare ecosystem. These will entail using AI techniques to create processors that can schedule doctor visits, gather medical data automatically, and decide which lab tests, prescription medications, and medical procedures to do. These groups might profit from more instruction in making decisions. NLP techniques can be used to analyze chaotic, non-digital data points in the construction of other classifiers. Test findings, physical examination notes, surgical notes, and other data relevant to patient discharge may be among them. Using historical data, machine learning may also be used to anticipate future events. It uses reinforcement learning, either uncontrolled or regulated, to forecast future occurrences.

8.3 APPLICATIONS OF IOMT IN POST-PANDEMIC MENTAL HEALTH CARE

The COVID-19 outbreak has spurred on the need for IoMT adoption in the mental health sector. The pandemic made it essential to incorporate remote examinations and follow-up in the delivery of care. With the aid of IoMT technologies, the shift toward virtual consultations and broader outreach by professionals has been made possible. In the post-epidemic landscape, IoMT continues to exert a transformative effect on the mental health care system. Easily accessible predictive IoMT combined with remotely delivered telepsychiatry enables real-time monitoring of various psychological parameters, thus helping provide early and personalized treatment, all of which stand to revolutionize care for each person. People will be able to manage their mental health with the help of the IoMT-based mobile application enhanced with various packages that include emotions tracking, virtual therapy sessions, and other assistance suited to the person's needs as a service. Emotions related to anxiety and trauma can be treated with immersion therapy which uses advanced therapeutic techniques such as virtual reality headsets and biofeedback devices. IoMT-equipped healthcare machines proactively analyze patients in order to identify illnesses and treat them in a way that avoids taking medication, or at the very least, makes it easier to maintain the effects of the medication. Furthermore, the technology assists caregivers by offering them education and additional communication tools. Post-pandemic, application of IoMT in mental health therapy can have better outcomes, improved access, and more personalization. Moreover, its ethical utilization should ensure the privacy concerns, security issues, and equity.

8.4 UTILIZING CODED LANGUAGE AND ALGORITHMS FOR DIAGNOSIS AND FOLLOW-UP

Mental health diagnosis and monitoring in IoMT comprises algorithms and programming languages. On top of that, IoMT can monitor data from multiple sources to detect trends and patterns to allow improved interventions and adjustments of treatment (Dinev & Hart, 2006). Using coded language and algorithms in mental health care (Hitchcock et al., 2022) represents enormous advancements in diagnosis accuracy, monitoring, and treatment progressions. By analyzing giant datasets containing known patterns of language, behavioral signs, and physical responses, advanced algorithms will allow healthcare providers to learn minute signals that may point to a mental health issue (Doryab et al., 2019). All of these types of data, from text messages to social media use to electronic health records (EHRs) to voice patterns captured during teletherapy sessions, can be analyzed by algorithms. The information from such input will yield coding advancement outcomes that will be advantageous to both the clients or patients and healthcare service providers (Hornstein et al., 2021).

Through natural language processing techniques, algorithms analyze the organization of text semantically and syntactically in order to identify hidden feelings, cognitive biases, and mental models that could indicate a mental health disorder (Chancellor et al., 2020).

Now, the algorithms applied in determining the overall tone of emotional connotation of any written or spoken communication might also capture any changes of mood or fluctuation that signals a possible shift in the mental health status (Torous et al., 2020). This enables the swifter identification of symptoms in their early stages and would allow for early intervention to prevent a crisis worsening (Shatte et al., 2019). The second potential breakthrough is that algorithms may uncover linguistic signatures of specific mental health disorders such as manic logorrhea, anxious avoidance, or depressive ruminations that guide the differential diagnosis and therapeutic planning (Keerthika et al., 2023). Algorithms in programming languages aid in customizing plans and interventions to an individual patient's specific traits, as well as their responses to treatment (Van Mens et al., 2023).

Algorithms can identify aspects that might be able to predict the likelihood of effective treatment results based on patterns in the analysis of patient data (Hornstein et al., 2021b) This information is then utilized to choose treatments that are empirically evidence-based and specific to the needs of individual patients (Gan et al., 2021). Algorithms can also generate personalized feedback and provide self-management recommendations. Patients can be proactive in their care due to this (Leong et al., 2021). Without an iota of doubt, the use of coded language and algorithms in mental health services has very serious ethical implications (Bipeta, 2019). Issues of data privacy, informed consent, algorithmic bias, and others must be addressed so that these technologies are used morally and responsibly (Obermeyer et al., 2019).

Besides the steps focused on protecting patient privacy and confidentiality, there is also a need to be open in communicating how patients' data will be collected and used. In addition, it is crucial to formulate and implement algorithms that minimize the effects of biases so that any decision-making would be just to stop disparities in treatment outcomes and access to healthcare (Torous et al., 2020). Applying this integration of algorithm and programming language could revolutionize monitoring and diagnosis in the post-pandemic age of mental health. Healthcare providers would integrate evidence-based insights, along with personalized treatments, to enable them to work more effectively, efficiently, and patient-centered.

8.5 TELECONSULTATION AND CODE CONSULTATION FOR MENTAL HEALTH

Teleconsultation and coding consultation through websites and applications have become widespread in the mental health treatment arena, especially since the epidemic. These systems ensure continuation of treatment as clinicians can remotely access clients and advise on light and medium situations. Teleconsultation and coded consultation are two innovative ways of expanding access to mental health services and promoting cooperation among practitioners in the area. The above technologies are of great benefit to both patients and healthcare providers, especially in the post-pandemic era where there is increased reliance on remote interactions. Teleconsultation is the delivery of clinical services through telecommunication technology. It includes assessments, treatment sessions, and medication prescription as part of mental health care. This methodology ensures easier access to mental health care by removing stigmatizing issues, geographical limitations, and other barriers related to transport.

Individuals are able to interact with mental health professionals from the comfort of their homes, through secure videoconferencing, thus encouraging timely interventions and streamlined care coordination. On the other hand, code consulting is a collaboration of mental health professionals in dealing with complex cases or clinical issues. An interdisciplinary approach can be used by medical professionals to share knowledge, seek additional perspectives, and develop innovative treatment plans that enhance the standard of patient care. Digital platforms and secure messaging services allow mental health practitioners to engage in real-time discussion forums, share clinical insights, and gain information from specialists in various fields. The benefits that accrue to teleconsultation and code consultation are significantly amplified when these two approaches are used in conjunction since this approach guarantees the most effective coordination of care and thereby increases the possibility of multidisciplinary collaboration. For example, a teleconsultation session involving a psychiatrist might include a code consultation involving a psychologist or a social worker; in this way, an integrated treatment plan for a patient suffering both mental and bodily health problems simultaneously may be designed.

Teleconsultation systems may also facilitate multidisciplinary team meetings with various medical specialists to deliberate on the complex needs of patients afflicted with severe mental illness or disease due to trauma. Teleconsultation, code consultation, and more judicious use of resources can also be helpful in allowing mental health care services to increase in scope and effectiveness, and other benefits like shorter waiting periods and more effective bureaucratic procedures. Healthcare institutions may utilize digital technology in improving accessibility, optimizing the coordination of care, and tailoring the treatment to the various needs of different patients in many settings, ranging from primary care locations to workplaces, educational institutions, and community centers. There are several factors that must be taken into consideration for the efficient implementation of teleconsultation and code consultation in the field of mental health care. These include patient privacy and confidentiality, compliance with legal requirements and licensing requirements, integration of telehealth platforms with EHRs, and supporting physicians in embracing collaborative and distant care models through support and training.

Teleconsultation and code consultation are potential game changers in the post-pandemic age to change the delivery of mental health treatment. Such modalities may increase access to high-quality care, encourage care integration, and enhance outcomes for people with mental health disorders through the use of technology and multidisciplinary teamwork.

8.6 NATURAL LANGUAGE PROCESSING IN MENTAL HEALTH ASSESSMENT

In evaluating individuals' mental status, there is involvement of NLP with its tools that use other sources, including medical records and social media, by applying the ability to draw value out of the information that appears within text to provide insight besides other conventional assessments used like mental status examination.

Applications of AI in IoMT include ML and NLP for e-healthcare. There are several uses of NLP and ML in e-healthcare clinical documentation discharge summaries and doctor's notes are examples of unstructured clinical documents from which NLP can automatically extract information. Following this, the algorithms of ML might analyze such information to establish patterns, extract relevant information, and append such details to the clinical databases or EHRs. In addition to the time and human labor involved in physically posting such information, this analysis enhances the dependability of clinical record-keeping. *Medical billing and coding:* The work of assigning appropriate medical codes for patients' conditions diagnosed, treatments they receive, or procedures they encounter can be automated using NLP and ML algorithms (Singh et al., 2023). These algorithms find an exact fit of the details captured in clinical notes and other relevant information with correct billing codes by reading through clinical notes and other pertinent data. This reduces error percentages and makes the process of coding and billing seamless. NLP- and ML-based patient data and medical literature analytics guide medical decisions regarding therapy advice. These algorithms can read diagnostic test results, extract information from medical literature, and make suggestions to doctors with solid evidence. It provides a more accurate prognosis and makes the treatment plan easy, ensuring that the best practices are used. The design of chatbots and virtual assistants in the healthcare sector is purely based on NLP and ML. These conversational agents can make an appointment, provide simple medical information, and provide users with personalized health advice, interpret, and respond to questions presented in natural language. With machine learning approaches, these systems could improve responses from users over time and adapt to individual preferences.

8.7 IOMT FACILITATING PSYCHOTHERAPEUTIC INTERVENTIONS

With IoMT technologies, real-time data and insights can be provided to professionals to make interventions in psychotherapy more effective. Improving the outcome of behavioral therapy designed for children as well as interpersonal psychotherapy targeted for adults are just examples. Psychotherapy practice is now changing due to IoMT technologies with their ability to enhance access, personalization, and efficacy through the use of connected devices. Through IoMT, psychotherapy therapies will finally reach remote places or other depressed areas by breaking the barriers of time and space and by offering real-time services. Biosensors designed for wearables will continuously measure physiological factors such as heart rate variability and electrodermal activity so that objective data can be collected and treatment planning together with response to a patient can be monitored. Another element of IoMT platforms is devices, which can involve patients and make them learn self-observation and self-regulation abilities. Virtual therapeutic environments, such as virtual reality exposure treatment for anxiety disorders or virtual mindfulness sessions for stress reduction, can also make patients participate in fully immersive psychotherapy experiences. These treatments offer a safe, controlled environment to facilitate an individual in working through psychological distress and achieving therapeutic objectives. Furthermore, with psychoeducation, self-help tools, and coping skill development by using interactive elements, IoMT-based mobile applications enable the patients to stay in control of their mental well-being between sessions. Another feature that IoMT provides is that it enables the conducting of telepsychiatry sessions. This means people can be treated from their homes.

With virtual consultations, mobility-related barriers of transportation and stigma are eliminated. Furthermore, asynchronous communication in IoMT systems with clients and therapists allows for constant support and guidance between sessions. However, in the wake of these advancements, ethical issues about data privacy, security, and the limits of therapy in the context of IoMT use must be duly considered. In addition, there is a need for further research in assessing the feasibility, acceptability, and effectiveness of IoMT-based treatments in various clinical settings and among diverse populations. When all these points are considered, IoMT could revolutionize psychotherapy by leveraging technology to make access, effectiveness, and participation in mental health care easier.

8.8 CASE STUDIES AND RESEARCH EVIDENCE

Based on the case studies and findings from this study, IoMT is quite promising in treatment for mental health conditions. Results have indicated effectiveness in IoMT-based treatments on improving the results of treatment, while revolutionizing the culture within the provision of mental health care.

Internet of Medical Things has introduced a new era in mental health care, providing unprecedented opportunities to improve patient outcomes, increase accessibility, and transform the delivery of medication. This chapter examines the transformative potential of IoMT in the treatment of mental health by analyzing implications and effectiveness based on case studies and empirical research data. Now, with the spread of digital technology, the continuous growth of connected devices has made it easy to fit IoMT into various branches of treatment for mental health, such as remote monitoring, tailored therapies, and collaborative care models. Mental health providers can use IoMTs to direct the treatment decision-making process by data-driven insights, predict outcomes, and personalize the therapies, meeting the different individual patient needs.

Numerous case studies have been presented that reflect the efficiency of IoMT therapy in mental health care. For example, by integrating biosensor-enabled wearable devices to monitor physiological anxiety-related symptoms, symptom reductions were highly achieved among individuals suffering from generalized anxiety disorder. Telepsychiatry service platforms also opened up avenues of mental health intervention for populations who were traditionally located in remote and rural settings. It further helped increase treatment response rates and compliance rates. Furthermore, VRET has proved to be beneficial in working with PTSD as it offers structured and immersive settings for therapeutic applications. Empirical evidence confirms the benefits of the Internet of Medical Things in delivering mental health care as it is embraced. From meta-analyses, telepsychiatry interventions promote the reduction of disparities in treatment outcomes and accessibility, especially to vulnerable populations. Besides that, the research has shown that there is an advantageous adoption of IoMT-enabled treatment for applications involving the identification of mental health symptoms, emergency forecasting, and personalization of treatment protocols.

This development brings along some implications for future action plans that cut across the lines of both practice and research. Through teleconsultation and remote monitoring, it makes it possible to give evidence-based treatments that are customized for each patient's requirements. It also promotes multidisciplinary teamwork and improves the patient–provider connection. However, questions about data privacy, security, and ethics must be addressed in order to guarantee that IoMT technologies are used in an ethical and responsible manner.

The Internet of Medical Things refers to the paradigm shift in delivering mental health treatment by offering revolutionary prospects for advancing patient-centered care, effectiveness, and accessibility. Mental health professionals can fully harness the opportunity of IoMT to meet new demands faced by individuals who are suffering from mental health problems and help transition the field toward a more connected and integrated future through findings from research and information from case studies.

8.9 FUTURE DIRECTIONS AND TRANSFORMATIVE CULTURE IN MENTAL HEALTH CARE

IoMT will increasingly play a significant role in the delivery of mental health care. Future research should focus on optimizing IoMT technologies, expand access to underserved populations, and address ethical and privacy concerns to realize the full potential of IoMT in promoting psychological well-being.

The changing culture and future directions defined by rising technology present a lot of prospective opportunities for innovation and development in the treatment of mental health. This chapter explores how the field of mental health treatment is changing and the revolutionary culture that patient-centered care and technological breakthroughs have produced:

- *Integration of Digital Health Technology:* The delivery of mental health treatment is set to be transformed by the integration of digital health technology, such as wearables, smartphone applications, and telehealth platforms. In the near future, these technologies will enhance patient participation by providing treatments tailored to the patient's needs, increasing access to care, and allowing for remote monitoring and interventions.
- *Data-Driven Insights and Predictive Analytics:* There is significant promise in treating mental illness by using predictive analytics and data-driven insights. Big data analytics and machine learning algorithms will allow practitioners in the area of mental health to see trends, predict outcomes, and personalize treatments based on patient characteristics and reactions to the treatment. All this will shape future treatment in order to get better results and prevent catastrophes while taking a proactive approach and preventionist way of treating mental health disorders.
- *Virtual and Augmented Reality Interventions:* The use of virtual and augmented reality is changing how mental health is approached. Further streams include the development and application of immersive technology in the provision of exposure therapy in PTSD, anxiety disorders, and phobias. Virtual reality environments create a safe and controlled environment for conducting therapy sessions in which individuals may confront and overcome psychological barriers within a safe and engaging environment.
- *Interdisciplinary Collaboration and Person-Centered Care:* The two underpinnings of the transformative culture in the treatment of mental

illness are person-centered care and interdisciplinary collaboration. In order to provide holistic, coordinated care, future models need to work toward establishing partnerships among mental health providers, primary care providers, social workers, and community agencies. Person-centered approaches make individuals' needs, values, and preferences a first priority and allow them to assume a leading role in the care and choices of their treatment.

- The first most important place for future improvement in mental health treatment is providing solutions to reducing inequity through equity. Overcoming barriers like stigma, barriers to access to care, as well as inadequate unequal distribution of healthcare resources toward everybody will prove the way out for ensuring their effective and quality-reached mental treatments. The help of culturally competent care, community-based interventions, and telehealth programs can help fill gaps in care and promote equity in mental health outcomes.

Transformational culture and technological breakthroughs will shape the future of mental health treatment, focusing on the use of digital health solutions, data-driven insights, immersive therapies, multidisciplinary cooperation, and equity-driven methods. In a rapidly changing world, mental health treatment can adapt to the changing needs of individuals and communities by embracing innovation and promoting a culture of continuous improvement.

Integration of IoMT in intellectual health care has the ability to absolutely rework and comply with diagnostic and treatment protocols, bringing a paradigm trade in the discipline. The use of IoMT technology enables intellectual healthcare experts to improve results from treatments, deliver custom-designed treatments, and make certain that remedy reaches all sufferers. Similarly, study and innovation on this vicinity are required for complete attainment of the benefits of IoMT. Hollis et al.'s (2017) studies show that telepsychiatry treatments can improve treatment effects and decrease inequalities in getting entry to intellectual healthcare, particularly for marginalized groups. In a comparable manner, Titov et al.'s meta-evaluation from 2019 proved the effectiveness of IoMT-enabled treatments in identifying mental health signs and symptoms, predicting crises, and tailoring treatment plans, such as sentiment analysis and predictive analytics. Within the context of the shipping of mental fitness care, studies by Gao et al. (2020) and Topol (2018) have established transformational capability for IoMT. It is pushing ahead the adherence to remedy, enhancing entry to care, and accordingly, patient outcomes. The findings here illustrate the vital significance of IoMT to the evolving needs of people with mental health disorders. IoMT holds a promise in influencing the character of intellectual fitness care shipping with probabilities for individualized remedies, advanced get right entry to care, and greater useful remedy outcomes. Ensuring that suitable and equitable adoption of IoMT technologies happens will require information privacy, security, and ethical concerns to be addressed. The integration of IoMT within the mental health area represents a brand-new paradigm, holding promise for modern diagnosis, treatment, and compliance with methods. Through the harnessing of technologies from IoMT, mental fitness companies can offer character-targeted interventions to enhance remedy effectiveness and make certain admission to care for all and sundry. In addition, studies and innovation can be necessary for the total recognition of the contributions IoMT can make to psychological well-being. The future prospects of IoMT in intellectual health treatment can simply be realized if there is steady funding for research and innovation. This will make it viable to develop proof-based plans for enforcing it inside the clinical practice surroundings. We are able to absolutely realize the ability of IoMT in enhancing psychological well-being of people.

REFERENCES

Bipeta, R. (2019). Legal and ethical aspects of mental health care. *Indian Journal of Psychological Medicine*, *41*(2), 108–112. https://doi.org/10.4103/ijpsym.ijpsym_59_19

Chancellor, S., & De Choudhury, M. (2020). Methods in predictive techniques for mental health status on social media: a critical review. *Npj Digital Medicine*, *3*(1). https://doi.org/10.1038/s41746-020-0233-7

Dinev, T., & Hart, P. (2006). An extended privacy calculus model for E-Commerce transactions. *Information Systems Research*, *17*(1), 61–80. https://doi.org/10.1287/isre.1060.0080

Doryab, A., Villalba, D. K., Chikersal, P., Dutcher, J. M., Tumminia, M., Liu, X., Cohen, S., Creswell, K., Mankoff, J., Creswell, J. D., & Dey, A. K. (2019). Identifying behavioral phenotypes of loneliness and social isolation with passive sensing: statistical analysis, data mining and machine learning of smartphone and fitbit data. *JMIR Mhealth and Uhealth*, *7*(7), e13209. https://doi.org/10.2196/13209

Gan, D. Z. Q., McGillivray, L., Han, J., Christensen, H., & Torok, M. (2021). Effect of engagement with digital interventions on mental health outcomes: A systematic review and meta-analysis. *Frontiers in Digital Health*, *3*. https://doi.org/10.3389/fdgth.2021.764079

Gao, J., Zheng, P., Jia, Y., Chen, H., Mao, Y., Chen, S., Wang, Y., Fu, H., & Dai, J. (2020). Mental health problems and social media exposure during COVID-19 outbreak. *PLOS ONE, 15*(4), e0231924. https://doi.org/10.1371/journal.pone.0231924

Gates, Lana. (2024). Future of healthcare: Internet of medical things. *Insight*, 23. January. https://mobilena.insight.com/en_US/content-and-resources/2021/future-of-healthcare-internet-of-medical-things.html

Hitchcock, P. F., Jr., Fried, E. I., & Frank, M. J. (2022). Needs time and context. *Annual Review of Psychology, 73*, 243–270. https://eiko-fried.com/wp-content/uploads/hitchcock-fried-frank-2022_final-published_annurev-psych-021621-124910.pdf

Hollis, C., R. Morriss, J. Martin, S. Amani, R. Cotton, M. Denis, et al., … Technological Innovations in Mental Healthcare Collaboration. (2017). Technological innovations in mental healthcare: Harnessing the digital revolution. *The British Journal of Psychiatry, 211*(4), 236–238. https://doi.org/10.1192/bjp.bp.116.195541

Hornstein, S., Forman-Hoffman, V., Nazander, A., Ranta, K., & Hilbert, K. (2021). Predicting therapy outcome in a digital mental health intervention for depression and anxiety: A machine learning approach. *Digital Health, 7*. https://doi.org/10.1177/20552076211060659

Joyce, D., De Brún, A., Mulcahy Symmons, S., Fox, R., & McAuliffe, E. (2023). Remote patient monitoring for COVID-19 patients: Comparisons and framework for reporting. *BMC Health Services Research, 23*(1) (3 August). https://doi.org/10.1186/s12913-023-09526-0

Keerthika, M., Abilash, K., Sundararaj Vasanth, M., Kuralamudhu, M. K., & Abbirooban, S. (2023). Emotional AI: Computationally intelligent devices for education. In *Elsevier eBooks* (pp. 87–99), 25 August. https://doi.org/10.1016/b978-0-443-19096-4.00007-9

Leong, Q. Y., Sridhar, S., Blasiak, A., Tadeo, X., Yeo, G., Remus, A., & Ho, D. (2021). Characteristics of mobile health platforms for depression and anxiety: Content analysis through a systematic review of the literature and systematic search of two app stores. *Journal of Medical Internet Research*, *24*(2), e27388. https://doi.org/10.2196/27388

Mathkor, D. M., Mathkor, N., Bassfar, Z., Bantun, F., Slama, P., Ahmad, F., & Haque, S. (2024). Multirole of the Internet of Medical Things (IoMT) in biomedical systems for managing smart healthcare systems: An overview of current and future innovative trends. *Journal of Infection and Public Health, 17*(4), 559–572. https://doi.org/10.1016/j.jiph.2024.01.013

Obermeyer, Z., Powers, B., Vogeli, C., & Mullainathan, S. (2019). Dissecting racial bias in an algorithm used to manage the health of populations. *Science*, *366*(6464), 447–453. https://doi.org/10.1126/science.aax2342

Patle, Divya Prabhudayal. 2024. Ontology based security recommendation for the Internet of Medical Things. *International Journal of Advance Research in Computer Science and Management Studies, 12*(7) (1. July), 321–329. https://doi.org/10.61161/ijarcsms.v12i7.40

Shatte, A. B. R., Hutchinson, D. M., & Teague, S. J. (2019). Machine learning in mental health: A scoping review of methods and applications. *Psychological Medicine*, *49*(09), 1426–1448. https://doi.org/10.1017/s0033291719000151

Singh, S., Joshi, R., Jain, P., & Abilash, K. (2023). Human AI: Ethics and broader impact for mental healthcare. In *Elsevier eBooks* (pp. 191–212). 25 August. https://doi.org/10.1016/b978-0-443-19096-4.00005-5

Topol, E. J. (2018). High-performance medicine: the convergence of human and artificial intelligence. *Nature Medicine*, *25*(1), 44–56. https://doi.org/10.1038/s41591-018-0300-7

Torous, J., Myrick, K. J., Rauseo-Ricupero, N., & Firth, J. (2020). Digital mental health and COVID-19: Using technology today to accelerate the curve on access and quality tomorrow. *JMIR Mental Health*, *7*(3), e18848. https://doi.org/10.2196/18848

Van Mens, K., Lokkerbol, J., Wijnen, B., Janssen, R., De Lange, R., & Tiemens, B. (2023). Predicting undesired treatment outcomes with Machine Learning in Mental Health Care: Multisite study. *JMIR Medical Informatics*, *11*, e44322. https://doi.org/10.2196/44322

9 Internet of Medical Things–Based Smart System for the Mental Health Care Challenges in 21st Century

Trends and Progress

Sreeja Gangadharan P., Abraham Francis, and Marsha Rodrigues

9.1 BACKGROUND

A healthcare system well connected to a collection of electronic devices and applications through an online computer system is Internet of Medical Things (IoMT). Such interconnected systems and health applications have a growing demand in the public healthcare domain due to the demand for ubiquitous computing in healthcare applications. A large number of remotely located devices or equipment can be connected in such an interconnected system, via the Internet or Wi-Fi. Applying AI to mental health care could expand access to mental health services to underserved communities and reduce costs and challenges involved in providing timely and quality services. This study reviews the applications of IoMT-based smart systems to effectively manage depression, a global "epidemic", and the related mental health care challenges in the present world.

9.2 DEPRESSION IN THE PRESENT WORLD

According to the WHO (2001), one in every four families have at least one member who is in need of mental health services. Across the world more than 500 million people suffer from mental health disorders, and it has become the most serious global health problem in the present world. Considering the world population, this is a huge number and there is an overwhelming majority of people who do not receive any treatment or receive inadequate treatment.

DOI: 10.1201/9781003476344-9

Depression is a common psychiatric disorder (WHO, 2017). Around 5% of the adult population across the world suffers from depression (WHO, 2023) making it a new silent epidemic globally. In a world where depression has become the leading cause of disability (Hadzic, 2008) and the factors that contribute to depression are rising on a day-to-day basis, it is essential that the mental health professionals should seriously look into all the possible ways to address this "epidemic."

Depression is characterized by diminished interest or pleasure in most or all activities, significant weight loss (or poor appetite) or weight gain, insomnia or hypersomnia, psychomotor retardation, fatigue or loss of energy, feelings of worthlessness or excessive or inappropriate guilt, diminished ability to think, concentrate or indecisiveness, recurrent thoughts of death, suicidal ideation, plan or attempt (DSM-5).

Lifestyle and environmental factors contribute to many mental health issues including depression. The adverse impacts associated with urbanization, increased competition, income disparity, political instability, economic crisis, changing family structure and nature of relationships, impact of AI and high-end technology, wars, and climate change have an enormous impact on the human race (Patel et al., 2018; Gilbert et al., 2009). Over the course of a few years, a surge in the amount of screen time with reduced exposure to natural environments have been observed (Balanzá-Martinez & Cervera-Martinez, 2022), and studies have established its relation with depression. The risks like extreme hot and unconducive environments to live in, unpredictable weather patterns, natural disasters, loss of life and property, are also making our life more miserable.

Scientists are coming up with new phenomena like the triple whammy effect which makes the planet earth unfit for living beings like humans and other beings in the near future. With the record temperature in every summer and the challenges it brings in our day-to-day life, we all are witnessing and receiving the negative impacts of these changes. Such changes in the environment on a large scale adversely affect our mental health and contribute to stress, depression, and anxiety. Studies on the nature of social media posts have stated that mental health and well-being of individuals worsen during warmer weather with these environmental factors affecting sleep, serotonin levels, medical inconsistency, and increased substance abuse (UCLA, 2023). In correlational studies using large sample, higher ambient temperature have been associated with an increase in suicide rates (Kim et al., 2019).

DSM-5 assumes depression as a unidimensional construct where the symptoms are summed up to determine the presence or the absence of a major episode (DSM-5) (American Psychiatric Association, 2013). However, a two-factor model represented by somatic and non-somatic factors was proposed by Elhai and colleagues in 2012, suggesting a better fit than the unidimensional model. According to the model, the somatic factors include sleep difficulties (SD), poor concentration, fatigue, appetite or weight changes, and psychomotor agitation/retardation. Non-somatic factors are affective items such as depressed mood, anhedonia, feelings of worthlessness, and thoughts of death. Clustering of symptoms into somatic and affective facilitates better tracking and recording of symptoms using technology.

A study conducted in Ethiopia states that around 39.16% of severe psychiatric disorders were misdiagnosed (Ayano et al., 2021). The study also pointed toward schizoaffective disorder and depression being the most common misdiagnosed psychiatric disorders. Most of the doctors rely on the patients reports for depression, anxiety and substance use disorders without checking criteria (Alegría et al., 2008). This limited information causes disparities in diagnosis. By harnessing the capabilities of IoMT in information accumulation and processing, reduced errors in diagnosis may be achieved. Applying AI to mental health care could expand access to mental health services to underserved communities and to reduce costs and challenges involved in providing timely and quality services.

9.3 NEED FOR THE USE OF ICT AND IOMT IN MENTAL HEALTH CARE

IoMT makes use of the technology components and applications in the healthcare domain while using artificial intelligence (AI) and machine learning (ML) as the common framework for collecting and processing the data (Yadav et al., 2019). Applying AI to mental health care could expand access to mental health services to underserved communities and reduce costs and challenges involved in providing timely and quality services. This is beneficial in making decisions which have policy implications related to healthcare for a region or a community.

Research and innovations in the field of wireless health are developing rapidly. The application of nanomedicine- and nanotechnology-enabled devices revolutionized healthcare services. Nanorobots are used in the field for various functions such as actuation, sensing, manipulation, propulsion, signaling, and information processing at the nanoscale. It is capable of replacing damaged neurons in patients and can perform neural surgeries as well as surgeries of the brain, with a high success rate (Ahmad et al., 2016). The efforts to use distributed computing which base their outcomes mostly on long-term monitoring activity patterns of individuals for cognitive disabilities like Alzheimer's and Autism are also under progress.

From the perspective of relevance in mental health, use of sensors, wearable devices, and mobile applications facilitate collection of pertinent data from the patients. This can consist of self-reported data as well as data gathered through devices. This helps to reduce the barriers due to geographic boundaries, distance, time, and costs to a great extent in the healthcare sector. Since healthcare is a priority sector, digital technology has a tremendous power in transforming the sector in terms of providing better service and improving efficiency and effectiveness in its operations.

9.4 VIRTUAL ENVIRONMENTS TO FACILITATE TREATMENT AND MENTAL HEALTH CARE

IoMT can be divided into four layers: an environmentally aware layer collecting data from sensors or smart devices which are then processed in the second layer known as the gateway layer. The gateways consist of Bluetooth, Wi-Fi, RFID, NFC, Satellite, and ZigBee. (Dwivedi et al., 2022). The data is then transmitted to the third layer—the cloud service layer where the data is stored and computed. The final layer is termed as the function layer where applications are carried out (Huang et al., 2023).

The wearable physical devices and implanted devices extract biosignals from the body, facilitating recording of mental health state of the users (Gupta et al., 2021; Swapna et al., 2022). Presence of such systems helps in communicating time-sensitive information about the patients or the users to researchers who can establish the predictability of depression among individuals through IoMT (Daisy et al., 2021; Ranaware & Joshi, 2020; Thulasi et al., 2023). Researchers have assessed movement monitoring and vitals such as heart rate, temperature, general health, and nutrition status (Dwivedi et al., 2022) along with physical symptoms of mental health conditions including headaches, nausea, cramps, perspiration etc., which can be observed and analyzed through AI and IoMT (Gupta et al., 2021).

Some of the common symptoms of mental health issues which can be effectively targeted using wearable sensors are palpitations, sweating, tremors, muscle tension, dizziness, nausea, and hyperventilation. The sympathetic and parasympathetic activation associated with the stress response can be measured indirectly by sensing the electrodermal activity (EDA). The production of sweat by the sympathetic nervous system (SNS) activation by the human body, which is by itself a non-voluntary action, can be assessed with the insertion of EDA sensors. It is one of the few non-invasive measures of sympathetic arousal. Along with this another important vital signal that is controlled by both the SNS and parasympathetic nervous system (PSN) during their different control states is the heart rate (HR) and heart rate variability (HRV).

Healey and colleagues (2005) are the pioneers in using physiological sensors which assess ECG, electromyogram (EMG), skin conductivity (also known as EDA or galvanic skin response [GSR]), and respiration (through chest cavity expansion) to monitor stress. The researchers associate 97% accuracy in determining stress levels by measuring heart rate and skin conductivity at intervals of 5 minutes (Healey et al., 2005). However, the accuracy in detecting stress levels dropped to 81.82% in an everyday setting as compared to a lab setting (Han et al., 2020).

Another major concern is the overlap of risk factors and symptoms among depression, anxiety, and stress (Ramón-Arbués et al., 2020). Hence, in such cases it is desirable to be monitored through questionnaires and checklists. However, there is no doubt in the efficiency of such systems in monitoring the progress of a diagnosed patient. With the help of ML, it is also possible to understand the pattern of variability in physiological indicators among individuals with various mental health conditions.

Some of the popular built-in monitoring wearable devices available on the market are BioPatch™ HP (Zephyr Technology, Annapolis, USA), an FDA-approved device which is a gold standard to compare data obtained from the other devices regarding their accuracy on HRV (Cruz et al., 2015) and the EQ02 LifeMonitor, which is a multi-parametric ambulatory health monitoring equipment that correlates well with standard laboratory devices for all physiological measures. There are many other devices such as Fitbit wearables, Mi Band, Empatica, etc., which are designed to track patients with epilepsy, physical well-being, mental health, and respiratory infections. In all these cases, the constraints are in terms of either cost or accuracy. There is a need for more research to validate the consistency of readings from these devices.

9.5 REMOTE PATIENT MONITORING (RPM)

RPM is a non-invasive technology now commonly integrated into disease management strategies with the goal of improving healthcare decision-making by providing additional patient information to the healthcare professionals. It employs ways to collect data from an individual through invasive sensors, smartphones/PDAs, computerized systems, wearables, or questionnaires (Vegesna et al., 2017). Healthcare professionals may share health data with remotely based clinical experts for consultation, saving time and expenses for practitioners and patients.

The wearable devices can be placed on the body to monitor any particular physiological changes (respiratory rate sensors or blood pressure monitors). Under certain conditions, biosensor devices are also used for recording data from biological or chemical reactions (e.g., pulse oximeters or spirometers). With the use of a smartphone or PDA device (or associated software/application/text messaging), the data gathered from the patient will be transmitted to the physician/researcher who will monitor the patient remotely, where a physician or a nurse provides feedback to the patient regarding the remotely captured data. This data feedback loop is a critical component in ensuring high impact on patient health in RPM interventions (Logan et al., 2012). Especially in mental health care, this will help in improving the quality of life through activation of self-care behaviors.

Some of the challenges identified in the large-scale implementation of the RPM are in terms of cost of technology and infrastructure to monitor, training providers in the collection and interpretation of results, incorporating the remote patient data into routine clinical practice, and educating patients in the use of devices (Steinhubl et al., 2015). However, many controlled studies have identified that the cost of non-invasive technologies is more effective in the long-term use (Luley et al., 2014). Even for the short-term use, the cost can be addressed by using insured reusable devices. The training required for the users can also be kept very minimal by reducing the human intervention in terms of feeding the data from the devices to the system. Lack of a smart algorithm in combining the relevant data to make informed decisions is also a drawback; however, this can be addressed by a dedicated research team working in the area of mental health and technology.

9.6 MEDICAL CYBER-PHYSICAL SYSTEMS (MCPS)

MCPS is an umbrella term for devices and software integrated in the healthcare domain, which works to provide better safety and care (Watson et al., 2022) by improving patient outcomes. It is a framework which combines embedded software control devices, networking capabilities, and complex physiological dynamics of patients in the modern medical field. The medical big data collected through the system provides great value in the areas of diagnosis, pathological analysis, epidemic tracking, pharmaceuticals, insurance, and so on (Chen et al., 2022). This framework accommodates many hard real-time health sensing devices, health diagnosis devices, and the user space composed of different users who provide information to the cyberspace. This cyberspace is the neural center of MCPS, which receives the sensing information from the physical space through the network transmission systems. It identifies, stores, analyses, and processes the information and generates the feedback which is sent to the physical space through a network transmission system (Chen et al., 2022).

The architecture can incorporate specific components to take care of the safety aspects. Therefore, every bit of information stored in the database will be kept safe from intrusion attempts (Alzahrani et al., 2023). It has varied applications for medical treatment in various venues such as home, office, school, or community. CPSs can positively impact the society, the economy, the environment, and individual citizens.

9.7 AUGMENTED ENVIRONMENT

Virtual reality (VR) and augmented reality (AR) can be used in therapeutic environments through effective amalgamation of distraction, extinction learning, cognitive-behavioral principles, gate-control theory, and spotlight theory of attention. In VR technology, modified reality experiences are provided to the users through a wearable head-mounted display (HMD) with a close-proximity screen that provides a "transported to three-dimensional life-like world" feeling. Evidence says that VR is effective in improving emotional well-being among cancer patients (Chirico et al., 2016). It can also be effectively used for anxiety disorders and pain management. In AR, superimposed computer images manipulate the users' view of the real world (Birckhead et al., 2019). The AR can be used as an effective training tool to deal with post-traumatic stress disorder (PTSD), anxiety and depressive symptoms. AR usage for reducing PTSD has been carried out for which the reduction rates observed ranges between 15% and 67% (Bhui, 2017; Yadav et al., 2019).

Hence, AR can be integrated to the IoMT-enabled therapeutic settings to provide real-time interventions and also to monitor the behavioral and physiological changes in the clients remotely. Usage of AR applications merged with IoMT sensors and ML for mental health rehabilitation help in predicting effective interventions and treatment while simultaneously reducing the burden on healthcare workers at hospitals and medical institutions.

9.8 CHALLENGES AND LIMITATIONS

The area of mental health assessment and diagnosis emphasize on both qualitative and quantitative information. "Dependence" on systems such as IoMT causes higher reliance to be placed on quantitative information and reduces focus on the narratives and relative experiences of the patients. Moreover, while the system has been proposed as useful to patients, clients, researchers and healthcare workers, overload of data may give rise to false predictions and reduce the scope for efficient management and interpretation of the data. Inaccurate readings, quality, and accuracy of the data may interfere with the efficiency of the system (Mathkor et al., 2024).

"Privacy" and "security" of the users is a major concern. Due to the pervasive nature of the system and its unfamiliar structure to the public, the users may not completely understand the process while agreeing to the data to be collected from them. Data leaks and breaches due to cybersecurity threats pose dangers to user identification and safety. Investing in technology such as IoMT for mental health is highly "expensive" and requires "familiarizing" yourself with the tech. Further resources such as equipment, expertise etc., in the area proves to be costly from a research perspective. To maintain efficiency, continuous validation of the results must take place which is challenging.

9.9 CONCLUDING REMARKS

Most of the doctors rely on the patients reports on depression, anxiety and substance use disorders without checking criteria (Alegría et al., 2008) and limited information causes disparities in diagnosis. By harnessing the capabilities of IoMT in information accumulation and processing can reduce errors in diagnosis. Using AI to promote better mental health of the population reduces the burden on the current system while attending to individuals who are in need of services the most. Internet of Things (IoT) and ML can be used to understand and predict the habitual activities of children (Masud et al., 2023), and their use in healthcare aids parenting in case of health emergencies or better monitoring and timely support. In the mental health domain, usage of such technology helps in carrying out timely intervention, preventing extreme outcomes by providing real-time alerts to the parents, guardians, caretakers, or therapists. Further, increased information improves the reliability of reciprocation between doctors and patients (Mathkor et al., 2024).

Around 150 million adults in India are in need of mental health care; however, they face the burden of accessibility. In an age where technology is prevalent and used by 66% of the global population and 75% of the population aged between 15 and 24 (Forbes, 2024), leveraging Internet access to enhance mental health care is not only relevant but highly essential. As there is an increase in developing healthcare applications worldwide, the IoMT market is said to reach an estimate of $158 billion in the United States. Since the market size of Indian healthcare is expected to grow at $372 billion (Dash, 2020) in the near future, increasing the potential for integrating technology with healthcare using IoMT is the need of the hour.

REFERENCES

Ahmad, U., & Faiyazudin, M. (2016). Smart nanobots: The future in nanomedicine and biotherapeutics. *Journal of Nanomedicine Biotherapeutic Discovery*, *6*(1). http://dx.doi.org/10.4172/2155-983X.1000e140

Alegría, M., Nakash, O., Lapatin, S., Oddo, V., Gao, S., Lin, J., & Normand, S. L. (2008). How missing information in diagnosis can lead to disparities in the clinical encounter. *Journal of Public Health Management and Practice: JPHMP*, *14*(Suppl), S26–S35. https://doi.org/10.1097/01.PHH.0000338384.82436.0d

Alzahrani, A., Alshehri, M., AlGhamdi, R., Sharma, S.K. (2023, January 29). Improved Wireless Medical Cyber-Physical System (IWMCPS) based on machine learning. *Healthcare* (Basel), *11*(3), 384. https://doi.org/10.3390/healthcare11030384

American Psychiatric Association. (2013). *Diagnostic and statistical manual of mental disorders* (5th ed.). Washington, DC. [Google Scholar] [Ref list]

Ayano, G., Demelash, S., Yohannes, Z., Haile, K., Tulu, M., Assefa, D., Tesfaye, A., Haile, K., Solomon, M., Chaka, A., & Tsegay, L. (2021). Misdiagnosis, detection rate, and associated factors of severe psychiatric disorders in specialized psychiatry centers in Ethiopia. *Annals of General Psychiatry*, *20*(1), 10. https://doi.org/10.1186/s12991-021-00333-7

Balanzá-Martínez, V., & Cervera-Martínez, J. (2022). Lifestyle prescription for depression with a focus on nature exposure and screen time: A narrative review. *International Journal of Environmental Research and Public Health*, *19*(9), 5094. https://doi.org/10.3390/ijerph19095094

Bhui, K. (2017). eHealth adventures in psychiatric therapeutics. *British Journal of Psychiatry*, *210*(4), 309–310. doi:10.1192/bjp.210.4.309

Birckhead, B., Khalil, C., Liu, X., Conovitz, S., Rizzo, A., Danovitch, I., Bullock, K., & Spiegel, B. (2019). Recommendations for methodology of Virtual Reality clinical trials in health care by an international working group: iterative study *JMIR Mental Health*, *6*(1). doi: 10.2196/11973

Chen, F., Tang, Y., Wang, C., Huang, J., Huang, C., Xie, D., Wang, T., & Zhao, C. (2022). Medical cyber–physical systems: a solution to smart health and the state of the art. *IEEE Transactions on Computational Social Systems*, *9*(5), 1359–1386. doi: 10.1109/TCSS.2021.3122807

Chirico, A., Lucidi, F., De Laurentiis, M., Milanese, C., Napoli, A., & Giordano, A. (2016). Virtual reality in health system: Beyond entertainment. A mini-review on the efficacy of VR during cancer treatment. *Journal of Cellular Physiology, 231*(2), 275–287. https://doi.org/10.1002/jcp.2511

Cruz, L., Rubin, J., Abreu, R., Ahern, S., Eldardiry, H., & Bobrow, D. G. (2015). *A wearable and mobile intervention delivery system for individuals with panic disorder.* Proceedings of the 14th International Conference on Mobile and Ubiquitous Multimedia, 175–182. ACM

Daisy, J., Kumar, B. V., & Krishnamoorthy, M. (2021). *Early-stage depression detector using IoMT.* International Conference on Advancements in Electrical, Electronics, Communication, Computing and Automation (ICAECA), 1–5. https://doi.org/10.1109/ICAECA52838.2021.9675629

Dash, S. P. (2020). The impact of IoT in healthcare: Global technological change & the roadmap to a networked architecture in India. *Journal of the Indian Institute of Science, 100*(4), 773–785. https://doi.org/10.1007/s41745-020-00208-y

Dwivedi, R., Mehrotra, D., & Chandra, S. (2022). Potential of Internet of Medical Things (IoMT) applications in building a smart healthcare system: A systematic review. *Journal of Oral Biology and Craniofacial Research, 12*(2), 302–318. https://doi.org/10.1016/j.jobcr.2021.11.010

Elhai, J. D., Contractor, A. A., Tamburrino, M., Fine, T. H., Prescott, M. R., Shirley, E., Chan, P. K., Slembarski, R., Liberzon, I., Galea, S., & Calabrese, J. R. (2012). The factor structure of major depression symptoms: A test of four competing models using the Patient Health Questionnaire-9. *Psychiatry Research, 199*, 169–173. https://doi.org/10.1016/j.psychres.2012.05.018

Forbes Home. (2024, March 1). *Internet usage statistics in 2024.* https://www.forbes.com/home-improvement/internet/internet-statistics/

Gilbert, P., McEwan, K., Bellew, R., Mills, A., & Gale, C. (2009). The dark side of competition: How competitive behaviour and striving to avoid inferiority are linked to depression, anxiety, stress and self-harm. *Psychology and Psychotherapy, 82*(Pt 2), 123–136. https://doi.org/10.1348/147608308X379806

Gupta, D., Bhatia, M. P. S., & Kumar, A. (2021). *Real-time mental health analytics using IoMT and social media datasets: Research and challenges.* Proceedings of the International Conference on Innovative Computing & Communication (ICICC) 2021. https://ssrn.com/abstract=3842818 or http://dx.doi.org/10.2139/ssrn.3842818

Hadzic, M., Chen, M., & Dillon, T. S. (2008). Towards the mental health ontology. Proceedings of the IEEE International Conference on Bioinformatics and Biomedicine. Philadelphia, PA.

Han, H. J., Labbaf, S., Borelli, J. L., Dutt, N., & Rahmani, A. M. (2020). Objective stress monitoring based on wearable sensors in everyday settings. *Journal of Medical Engineering & Technology, 44*(3), 177–189. https://doi.org/10.1080/03091902.2020.1759707

Healey, J. A., & Picard, R. W. (2005). Detecting stress during real-world driving tasks using physiological sensors. *IEEE Transactions on Intelligent Transportation Systems, 6*(2), 156–166. https://doi.org/10.1109/TITS.2005.848368

Huang, C., Wang, J., Wang, S., & Zhang, Y. (2023). Internet of medical things: A systematic review. *Neurocomputing, 557,* 126719. https://doi.org/10.1016/j.neucom.2023.126719

Kim, Y., Kim, H., Gasparrini, A., Armstrong, B., Honda, Y., Chung, Y., Ng, C. F. S., Tobias, A., Íñiguez, C., Lavigne, E., Sera, F., Vicedo-Cabrera, A. M., Ragettli, M. S., Scovronick, N., Acquaotta, F., Chen, B. Y., Guo, Y. L., Seposo, X., Dang, T. N., de Sousa Zanotti Stagliorio Coelho, M., … Hashizume, M. (2019). Suicide and ambient temperature: A multi-country multi-city study. *Environmental Health Perspectives, 127*(11), 117007. https://doi.org/10.1289/EHP4898

Logan, A. G., Irvine, M. J., McIsaac, W. J., Tisler, A., Rossos, P. G., Easty, A., Feig, D. S., & Cafazzo, J. A. (2012). Effect of home blood pressure telemonitoring with self-care support on uncontrolled systolic hypertension in diabetics. *Hypertension, 60*(1), 51–57. https://doi.org/10.1161/HYPERTENSIONAHA.111.188409

Luley, C., Blaik, A., Götz, A., Kicherer, F., Kropf, S., Isermann, B., Stumm, G., & Westphal, S. (2014). Weight loss by telemonitoring of nutrition and physical activity in patients with metabolic syndrome for 1 year. *Journal of the American College of Nutrition, 33*(5), 363–374. https://doi.org/10.1080/07315724.2013.875437

Masud, K. I., Shuvo, M. H., Al Mamun, A., Mallick, J., Jannat, M. R., & Rahman, M. O. (2023). Developing an IoT-based child safety and monitoring system: An efficient approach. In 2023 26th International Conference on Computer and Information Technology (ICCIT) (pp. 1–6). IEEE. https://doi.org/10.1109/ICCIT60459.2023.10441116

Mathkor, D. M., Mathkor, N., Bassfar, Z., Bantun, F., Slama, P., Ahmad, F., & Haque, S. (2024). Multirole of the Internet of Medical Things (IoMT) in biomedical systems for managing smart healthcare systems: An overview of current and future innovative trends. *Journal of Infection and Public Health, 17*(4), 559–572. https://doi.org/10.1016/j.jiph.2024.01.013

Patel, V., Burns, J. K., Dhingra, M., Tarver, L., Kohrt, B. A., & Lund, C. (2018). Income inequality and depression: A systematic review and meta-analysis of the association and a scoping review of mechanisms. *World Psychiatry, 17*(1), 76–89. https://doi.org/10.1002/wps.20492

Ramón-Arbués, E., Gea-Caballero, V., Granada-López, J. M., Juárez-Vela, R., Pellicer-García, B., & Antón-Solanas, I. (2020). The prevalence of depression, anxiety and stress and their associated factors in college students. *International Journal of Environmental Research and Public Health, 17*(19), 7001. https://doi.org/10.3390/ijerph17197001

Ranaware, M. V., & Joshi, K. (2020). Depression monitoring using wearable sensors. *Journal of Emerging Technologies and Innovative Research*. https://www.jetir.org/papers/JETIR2003391.pdf

Steinhubl, S. R., Muse, E. D., & Topol, E. J. (2015). The emerging field of mobile health. *Science Translational Medicine, 7*(283), 283rv3. https://doi.org/10.1126/scitranslmed.aaa3487

Swapna, M., Viswanadhula, U. M., Aluvalu, R., Vardharajan, V., & Kotecha, K. (2022). Bio-signals in medical applications and challenges using artificial intelligence. *Journal of Sensor and Actuator Networks, 11*(1), 17. https://doi.org/10.3390/jsan11010017

Thulasi, K., Balakrishnan, S., Tue, L., Monpreeyadee, R., Fatima, S. R., Rosli, M. I. S., Wei, G. Q., & Malarvili, M. B. (2023). *IoT-enabled wearable prototype: Detecting signs of depression*. Proceedings of the 2023 7th International Conference on Computational Biology and Bioinformatics (ICCBB), 1–6. ACM. https://doi.org/10.1145/3638569.3638580

UCLA Health. (2023, September 26). *Four effects of heat on mental health (and how to protect yourself)*. https://www.uclahealth.org/news/article/4-effects-heat-mental-health-and-how-protect-yourself-2

Vegesna, A., Tran, M., Angelaccio, M., & Arcona, S. (2017). Remote patient monitoring via non-invasive digital technologies: A systematic review. *Telemedicine and e-Health, 23*(1), 3–17. https://doi.org/10.1089/tmj.2016.0051

Watson, A., Park, J., Pugh, S., Sokolsky, O., Weimer, J., & Lee, I. (2022). *Medical cyber-physical systems: IoMT applications and challenges*. 2022 56th Asilomar Conference on Signals, Systems, and Computers, 998–1004. IEEE. https://doi.org/10.1109/IEEECONF56349.2022.10052004

World Health Organization. (2001). *The world health report 2001: Mental health—New understanding, new hope*. WHO. https://www.who.int/whr/2001/en/

World Health Organization. (2017). *World Health Day 2017—Depression: Let's talk*. https://www.who.int/news-room/events/detail/2017/04/07/default-calendar/world-health-day-2017

World Health Organization. (2023). *Depressive disorder (depression)*. https://www.who.int/news-room/fact-sheets/detail/depression

Yadav, N., Jin, Y., & Stevano, L. J. (2019). *AR-IoMT mental health rehabilitation applications for smart cities*. 2019 IEEE 16th International Conference on Smart Cities: Improving Quality of Life Using ICT & IoT and AI, 166–170. IEEE. https://doi.org/10.1109/HONET.2019.8907997

10 Healing beyond Beliefs

A Posthumanist Reading of IoMT Advancements

Jehoson Jiresh J., Abishek A., and Abarna SriPreethi K.

10.1 INTRODUCTION

The advent of Internet of Medical Things (IoMT) in healthcare is a transformative paradigm that drastically reshapes the healthcare paradigm. As an offshoot of the Internet of Things (IoT), it leverages interconnected medical devices, sensors, wearables, and systems to enhance patient care and clinical outcomes by ensuring effective collection, analysis, and exchange of health data (Al-Turjman et al. 2020, 644; Joyia et al. 2017, 240). It provides unparalleled opportunities for remote monitoring, early diagnosis, and bespoke treatment (Vishnu, Ramson, and Jegan 2020, 101). IoMT offers an enterprising platform for enhancing the quality of life while ensuring more cost-effective and efficient healthcare systems (Al-Turjman et al. 2020, 645; Srivastava et al. 2022). By ensuring real-time data transfer among patients, healthcare providers, and system databases, IoMT is projected to address crucial challenges in healthcare services, from enriching preventive care to effectuating and optimizing hospital treatments (Majeed, Nazir, and Schneider 2023, 129). Integrating IoMT with artificial intelligence (AI), blockchain, and big data analytics powered by a 5G network opens new avenues in medical research and personalized healthcare (Razdan and Sharma 2021, 775).

While the positive impact of IoMT in healthcare systems is undeniable, the point of discussion in this chapter is a sociocultural probe into the religious response to these technological endeavors. The interplay of religion and technology has historically been intricate and mostly contentious (Ahmed, Haseeb, and La 2021, 219). Despite IoMT's pathbreaking contribution to enhancing healthcare practices, it is contested by some solid religious convictions, beliefs, and practices. The religious resistance to specific technological advancements in healthcare, especially those involving IoMT devices, often arises from interpretations of sacred texts and age-old beliefs about the sanctity attributed to the human body, which goes against the intake or implant of anything artificial. In some instances, such implants are even viewed as the devil's scheme to gain control over humankind and the potential fulfillment of specific scriptural prophecies, thus making a call to the believers that to remain pure

DOI: 10.1201/9781003476344-10

and divine, one should abstain from taking any artificial implants in the body. For example, some Christians interpret the passage Revelation 13:16–18, which warns believers against receiving “the mark of the beast” to warn against implantable healthcare devices or other technologies that could be considered agents that alter the divinely created human body (Doyle 2017). However, over the years, the human need and inherent love to increase life expectancy through optimum healthcare have withstood the religious resistance to technological interventions to repair human healthcare conditions.

The resistance to technological progress in the form of religious beliefs is not limited to one specific religion but is found across various faith traditions. The authors argue that these concerns often revolve around human dignity, sanctity of life, holiness or purity, and limiting human intervention in what is understood as the natural or divinely ordained order. This phenomenon of faith attempting to limit human scientific endeavor is due to religions’ ever-fixated ideas on creation, preservation, and destruction of the world and the subsequent fear that the discoveries and inventions pioneered by scientific pursuits would contest the authority and authenticity of religious narratives. However, it is also vital to note that the relationship between religion and technology is not entirely antagonistic. Several religious traditions have historically supported technological and scientific endeavors, including medicine (Ahmed, Haseeb, and La 2021, 220).

In the present-day context, some religious factions and communities actively participate in discussions concerning the ethical challenges of novel medical technologies, attempting to wed with faith and scientific progress. At this juncture, as IoMT continues to expand and evolve its range in healthcare, negotiating these tensions will be vital. It requires continuous dialogue among healthcare providers, technologists, ethicists, religious leaders, and believers to discuss concerns and normalize scientific temper to encounter superstitions and pseudoscientific narratives. In addition, such deliberations are pertinent to democratize technological advancements among diverse groups of people to optimize the potential benefits of scientific advancements and ensure enhanced living conditions.

This chapter presents a discourse on normalizing the interplay between humans and technology using a posthumanist theoretical reading. The posthumanist approach provides a critical viewpoint to understand the blurring bounding between human and non-human entities. It also resonates with the significance of scientific interventions in informing cultural change, living standards, and healthcare and well-being. In addition, this chapter explores how IoMT blur the boundaries between humans and technology and encounters the religion-based and biased sociocultural resistance to these advancements. It also suggests ways to challenge such resistance using rationality and critical discussions, primarily by exposing the (un)conscious shift in belief systems, which is informed and influenced by scientific advancements. By facilitating such progressive discussions, the authors of this chapter argue that IoMT healthcare solutions can be normalized among the masses, which, in turn, will lead to the potential democratization of healthcare solutions to ensure accessibility and affordability.

10.2 THEORETICAL FRAMEWORK

The present discourse uses posthumanist theory to analyze the intricate interplay of humans, technology, and health in the context of the IoMT developments. Posthumanism per se contests traditional anthropocentric perspectives argues against the idea of having humans as the primary subject of any analysis and explores the complex relationships between humans, non-human entities, and technology (Buran et al., 2021, 1–2; Hayles, 1999). Several posthumanists have considerably reshaped our perception of the human condition in a technology-driven world. Donna Haraway's (1991) conceptualization of the "cyborg" envisions the interplay of humans and machines. Katherine Hayles (1999) opines that humans are already posthuman, emphasizing the imbricate network of human consciousness with digital technologies. On the same lines, Bruno Latour's (2005) actor–network theory offers an ontological understanding where humans and non-humans are equal actants in complex networks. Rosi Braidotti's (2013) ideation of the posthuman condition provides a favorable sociopolitical discourse, as quoted in Toffoletti, "combines critique with creativity in the pursuit of alternative visions and projects" (2015, 212).

The posthumanist approach is an apposite framework to analyze the sociocultural perception of IoMT, as it argues for moving beyond the traditional boundaries of human–technology negotiations. It inspires deliberation on how IoMT technologies are not only external tools but also integral symbols signifying the human experience of health and well-being. This approach facilitates the analysis of IoMT devices as active participants in the healthcare context, impacting diagnoses, treatment decision-making, and patient experiences. The utilitarian focus of posthumanism, as stated by Bakošová and Odorčák (2020, 47–62), fosters investigation of how IoMT devices physically interact with and effectively alter human bodies, blurring the lines between the natural or organic and the naturalized technological processes.

Furthermore, the posthumanist critique of human exceptionalism and anthropocentrism (Krupa 2021, 75–94) offers a valuable viewpoint to examine the ethical implications of IoMT. It kindles narratives on how these technologies might contest traditional beliefs of human and divine autonomy in healthcare diagnosis, decision-making, and probing of more distributed, democratized models of treatment in health management. Consequently, this chapter aims to venture beyond simplistic notions of technological progress or dystopian fears by employing a posthumanist theoretical framework. Thus, it seeks to provide a detailed analysis of how IoMT advancements are reframing and reimagining the healthcare landscape and effectively opening new possibilities for healing and well-being in a posthuman world.

10.3 DISCUSSION

The Internet of Medical Things refers to an interconnected network of smart devices, medical equipment, software applications, and healthcare systems that communicate and transfer data using the Internet (Huang et al. 2023). The interconnected network of IoMT realizes the posthumanist preposition of removing the human subject from the center, contesting anthropocentrism (Buran et al. 2021, 1–4; Hayles 1991).

The elements of IoMT involving wearable devices, remote monitoring systems, intelligent implants, sensors, actuators, software applications, cloud platforms, and network infrastructure (Sharma, Tomar, and Preeti 2022, 61) epitomize Katherine Hayles' (1999) postulation that humans are already posthuman, deeply connected with digital technologies and information systems. Today, these devices and systems are external tools intrinsic to the human healthcare experience, blurring the boundaries between the organic and the technological. The coaction of artificial intelligence and machine learning algorithms with IoMT systems (Wong et al. 2021, 427) resonates with Bruno Latour's (2005) actor–network theory, where humans and non-humans are considered equal actants in complex networks. These AI-powered networks examine large amounts of patient data in real time, identifying patterns and anomalies that might escape human observers, thus contesting human autonomy in healthcare diagnostics and decision-making.

The COVID-19 pandemic has quickened the exponential emergence of remote patient monitoring using IoMTs and telemedicine (Shakeel et al. 2023, 1027). The new normal actualized by this rapid shift reflects the posthumanist critique of human exceptionalism and anthropocentrism (Krupa 2021, 75–94). It, in turn, expands healthcare beyond conventional human-centric hospital contexts. Besides, it constructs a distributed network of care that involves the collaboration of human and non-human actors. As Akilan et al. (2023, 967) argued, smart healthcare facilities integrated this idea with interconnected devices and sensors, optimizing patient care and resource management and exhibiting how non-human players can effectively engage in and influence healthier ecosystems.

Considering this paradigm shift, it is evident that constant advancements in IoMT continue to reflect a posthumanist fervor depicting how a complex interplay of various organic and technological actors works in tandem to ensure health and well-being. Therefore, this chapter will further deliberate the following vital sociocultural aspects of IoMT using a posthumanist theoretical framework established earlier:

i. Transhumanist projects and posthumanism
ii. Blurring human and non-human boundaries
iii. Sociocultural religious resistance to IoMT
iv. Ethical implications and future directions

These sections will trace the relationship between IoMT developments and posthumanist ideations. However, the crucial point of discussion in this chapter encompasses a critical discourse on the sociocultural resistance to IoMT that sprouts from conventional beliefs, resulting in resistance to technology. Furthermore, this chapter discusses the ethical implications of such resistance and other ethical concerns, challenges, and opportunities in this ever-evolving medical landscape.

10.4 TRANSHUMANIST PROJECTS AND POSTHUMANISM

The IoMT emergence is a practical execution of transhumanist pursuits, manifesting posthumanist philosophy fostered by speciesist human interests. Transhumanism aims to enhance human capabilities, encompassing life expectancy and physical and mental capabilities, through pathbreaking innovations in genetic engineering, biotechnology, and AI (Devlin, 2014). These goals of transhumanism align with the objectives of IoMT, which strives to enhance health outcomes and expand human life through technological interventions. IoMT advancements contribute to these objectives by enabling continuous health monitoring, early detaching of diseases, diagnostics, and personalized treatment plans. For example, wearable devices that track vital parameters and force health risks (Huang et al. 2023) can be viewed as efforts to achieve the transhumanist vision of improving human biology.

In addition, integrating AI and ML in IoMT (Wong et al. 2021, 427) aligns with transhumanist ambitions of cognitive enhancement. An example of transhumanist accomplishments is the invention and introduction of neuralink, aimed at improving the quality of life among individuals with severe brain and spinal cord injuries by empowering them to access computers and other gadgets using their brain signals (Venkatesh et al. 2022, 389; Fiani et al. 2021). Such technologies supplement human decision-making in healthcare, other domains, and mundane human activities. As mentioned, these technologies facilitate enhanced diagnostic accuracy and treatment efficacy in healthcare. As IoMT technologies advance, they may progressively complement transhumanist pursuits with more considerable human interest.

10.5 BLURRING HUMAN AND NON-HUMAN BOUNDARIES

The amalgamation of IoMT devices with human bodies symbolized Donna Haraway's (1991) cyborg concept, surpassing the conventional limits of humans and machines. Implantable cardiac defibrillators, continuous glucose monitors, intelligent knee implants, and insulin pumps are seamlessly integrated with the human body (Sharma, Tomar, and Preeti 2022, 61–73). These hybrid entities contest conventional ideas of the "natural" human body. These devices monitor and intervene in bodily processes, making autonomous decisions that were once considered the realm of natural processes or, in religious narratives, divine intervention. Innovative advancements in brain–computer interfaces, thought-controlled robotic prosthetic limbs, and ingestible sensors (Vilela and Hochberg 2020, 87) elate our perception of complex human identity regarding its relationship between body and technology. Such innovations encapsulate Rosi Braidotti's (2013) affirmative politics, integrating critique with creativity to unravel new possibilities for rethinking healthcare practices and patient, treatment–provider relationships. The posthumanist approach enables critics to surpass simplistic narratives of technological progress or dystopian fears and offers a nuanced examination of how IoMT developments are reshaping the healthcare landscape. It ensures a shift in rereading the conventional understanding of technology's influence on human autonomy in healthcare decision-making and analyzes more distributed and relational agency models in health management.

10.6 SOCIOCULTURAL RESISTANCE TO IOMT

Since its introduction, integrating IoMT technologies has faced sociocultural resistance, especially from religious factions that view the human body as sacred and god-created (Fahmy 2022). These factions view IoMT tools as unnatural interventions in the divinely created human body (Doyle 2017). The religious resistance to IoMT and other healthcare technologies is rationalized using the following claims, identified by the authors based on their interactions with believers from different faiths:

i. Caution against implantable medical devices as they are viewed as potential means for the evil or the devil to control humans.
ii. Concerns against the potential of devices to alter the human body's naturalness are seen as tampering with the almighty divine's creation.
iii. The concept of karma and depicting the body as a temporary vessel and any technological intervention is viewed as an intervention that impedes the imaginary spiritual soul's eternal journey.

The reasons for resistance mirror the conflict between traditional anthropocentric or theocentric views and the posthuman reality of technology-driven healthcare. In most cases, resistance is fostered by "pastoral power" or the "government of souls" (Foucault 2007), a power form that interferes with people's lives, choices, and behavior to ensure salvation. However, the unquestionable necessity and advantages of IoMT have resulted in its gradual unconscious acceptance across diverse religious factions. Many believers have come to terms with reality, but by claiming that their god gives his people wisdom to develop and invent such technologies. Such claims may offer them a sense of satisfaction while reinstating god's role even in technology-driven pursuits.

The shift in spiritual narratives, beliefs, and practices is observed in the changing contents of prayers. Praying for miraculous healing is progressively accompanied by or substituted with prayers for accurate diagnosis and accessing the best medical treatment, which portrays an unconscious acceptance of scientific intervention as the ultimate solution and paves the way for the integration of faith and science. This shift portrays a form of amalgamation of faith and science, where supernatural interventions are requested not to avoid medical treatment but to bless and guard the patient during the treatment procedure involving advanced technologies. In some cases, rituals and blessings are organized before inaugurating hospitals, medical devices, and equipment and starting a medical procedure. Moreover, the shift exhibits the unconscious acceptance of the posthuman viewpoint that acknowledges the agency of non-human actors, in this context, IoMT technologies, in healthcare practices and results.

However, after listening to a few faith testimonies on "miraculous" healing, the authors argue that the tendency in accident and chronic disease survivors' testimonies to ascribe healing mainly to supernatural divine power instead of acknowledging the role of healthcare technology posits a challenge. Such narratives, which more often than not eclipse the complex medical process and technological interference facilitating recovery, can adversely influence the larger population and mislead them into relying entirely on faith healers rather than seeking timely scientific solutions. Ironically, the medical care beneficiaries fail to acknowledge the role of science and the economic stability that enabled them to acquire the treatment. Instead, they attribute healing to the "divine grace"; in some cases, even physicians impute divine intervention in the healing process. The authors of this chapter infer that this phenomenon is prevalent among physicians as a caveat put forth by medical practitioners to safeguard themselves from impending risks due to potential negligence, ignorance, and any other unforeseen circumstances during the treatment process. Reading such narratives using a posthumanist lens critically perceives these as narratives which propagate anthropocentric and theocentric views and fail to realize the intricate involvement of human and non-human actor networks in the healing process.

Similarly, popular beliefs that attribute life events to fate, an explanation to an event or occurrence as predestined, fail to acknowledge the role of IoMTs and other healthcare interventions in altering the predestined. Such simplistic explanations in most belief systems downplay the role of healthcare advancements in altering fate through accurate diagnosis and effective treatments. While writing this chapter, one of the authors encountered a real-life incident that exemplifies how fate-based and biased narratives can downplay the role of scientific development in healthcare. It eventually leads to a hopeless worldview where people live only to react and respond to the so-called destiny, stating, "It is not in our hands" to comfort themselves during distress. The incident revolves around the tragic death of an 18-year-old student at a university due to cardiac arrest. He was found dead alone in his rented apartment. The subsequent discussion among a few faculty members concluded that the boy's death could not be stopped as it was his fate, written in destiny.

The authors identify the following five factors as the reason behind attributing events to fate:

i. A cognitive dissonance, as scientific explanations can be complex and difficult to fathom. The dissonance arises due to a lack of scientific literature, leading to a fear of the unknown; scientific explanations reflecting unexpected aspects of life create anxiety.
ii. Narratives on fate and destiny ensure a sense of control as people believe that someone or something controls this universe and its events, which can be ironically comforting. It also provides an imaginary connection to something more significant, the universe or the so-called cosmic plan.
iii. The emotional solace the destiny narrative offers, especially during uncertainty and sorrow. It seemingly offers a sense of purpose and meaning.
iv. The environment determines cultural and social factors due to upbringing, tradition, peer pressure, and the fear of being typecast as abnormal or rebellious in a society that accepts fate as usual. As a result, such pseudoscientific beliefs, in many cases, have become habits.

v. Psychological prejudices such as anchoring bias, confirmation bias, and availability heuristic may favor destiny over scientific explanations.

However, after the conclusion locating fate as the reason for the sudden demise of the student, the author had to respond by stating that, a few centuries ago, any mysterious fever was considered an inescapable fate. Today, people usually intervene in such situations with simple medication or seek further diagnosis and treatment if the fever persists. Indeed, people do not leave it to fate anymore. This drastic shift in approach portrays how human intervention using healthcare advancements has efficiently "altered" or "postponed" what might have earlier been viewed as predestined. In addition, taking insights from the experience of working on this chapter, the author argued that the academic community should restrain from normalizing such ignorant, simplistic explanations. Instead, the educated lot should deliberate on ensuring accessibility to Internet-driven health monitoring systems to avoid such deaths in the future.

In the context of IoMT, wearable gadgets or health-tracking implants that monitor vital signs could alert emergency aid or individuals around in cases of sudden collapse. The day is near when emergency treatment from remote locations using IoMT becomes normal. As it stands, IoMT ensures constant, real-time monitoring of patient's vitals, enhancing the ability to diagnose and treat health conditions remotely. Wearable sensors and IoMT devices can acquire and transmit data to healthcare professionals, ensuring timely medical interventions (Syed et al. 2019, 101; Alshormanm O et al. 2020, 414; Subha et al. 2023, 1–6; Rashed et al. 2017, 160; Subramaniam et al. 2023; Khan et al. 2021). This real-life instance and the subsequent discourse underpin the significance of contesting dominant narratives of divine will and fate with scientific counternarratives to examine the interplay of human agency and technological intervention in healthcare. From a posthumanist lens, by blurring the boundaries between human entities and machine aid, a new paradigm evolves where vital life-defining biological factors are monitored and protected by interconnected devices.

On that account, to encounter the crucial challenge of resistance to technology, which impacts the masses from embracing scientific interventions in their healthcare journey, it is vital to popularize narratives that foreground medical interventions. The narratives on spiritual experience related to healing should be limited to acknowledging how it offered comfort and hope during distress. Promoting a comprehensive perception of the healing process will capture the essence of the posthuman condition. Fostering scientific temper, critical thinking, and evidence-based decision-making play vital roles in enabling people to embrace IoMT developments constructively. Normalizing such critical perspectives will primarily argue against human exceptionalism and encourage a more distributed understanding of healthcare agency that combines human and technological actants. Furthermore, by demonstrating the tangible outcomes and advantages of technology in healthcare, IoMT can construct a more informed and scientifically sensible society that is better poised to negotiate complex health issues. At this juncture, it is noteworthy to state that the COVID-19 pandemic has, to an extent, escalated the acceptance of medical technologies involving remote monitoring and telemedicine that were irreplaceable during the lockdown (Hegde and Eid 2021).

Along the same lines, effective policy frameworks and legal systems to check the unscientific healing processes and expose their vulnerability to the larger populace are equally important. Moreover, efforts to streamline the medical industry and make IoMT applications accessible and affordable to people are also crucial and pertinent. Effective democratization of wearable devices and remote monitoring systems can expand healthcare services to underserved sections of society, reducing disparities in access to healthcare. In this pursuit, it is vital to encounter the concerns of digital literacy and the digital divide to ensure equitable distribution of the benefits of IoMT. These earnest endeavors will unleash the potential of technology to eliminate existing inequalities and ensure empowerment. These initiatives align with the potential of IoMT to democratize healthcare by making advanced healthcare solutions accessible to people from various strata of society (Akilan et al. 2023, 972). Thus, it resonates with the posthumanist objective of challenging conventional boundaries and traditional hierarchies.

10.7 ETHICAL IMPLICATIONS AND FUTURE DIRECTIONS

The amalgamation of IoMT into healthcare evokes pertinent ethical considerations that bisect with posthumanist and transhumanist philosophies. Since these technologies become more profound and integrated with human bodies, questions arise concerning privacy, autonomy, and the naturalness of human identity. Data security and privacy are apposite concerns in the IoMT environment. The abundant personal health data collected and transmitted by these devices (Ghubaish et al. 2020, 8718) elicit questions about data ownership, consent, and the potential for surveillance, which resonates with arguments closely related to the discourse on biopower, possessing power over bodies (Foucault 1978). From a posthumanist viewpoint, such data transmission can be viewed as expanding the human self into the digital domain, blurring the boundaries between personal and public, human and machine. The autonomy of AI-driven IoMT devices in forming healthcare decisions contests conventional claims of human agency in healthcare contexts. As these systems have become more sophisticated, there can be occurrences where they form decisions that conflict with patients' cultural choices, beliefs, and customs. Such a context calls for a rethinking of healthcare ethics that resonates with the agency of non-human actors while prioritizing human well-being and autonomy.

The transhumanist facet of IoMT also invites questions about accessibility and equity. While these technologies have primarily improved human health and life expectancy, there is a risk of creating newer versions of inequality based on access to IoMT technologies. Guaranteeing equitable access to IoMT developments is vital to realizing their potential for enhancing global health indices. In the future, the persistent advancements of IoMT technologies will likely contest our perception of what it means to be human. As these devices are gradually becoming an integral part of human bodies and minds, it is germane to reconsider legal and ethical frameworks revolving around personhood, responsibility, and rights. For this reason, posthumanist reading offers a practical framework for navigating these complex concerns, encouraging humans to think beyond conventional human-centric discourses.

To ensure a healthy posthuman understanding of the IoMTs and other healthcare advancements, a cohesive coaction of the following aspects becomes imperative:

i. Enriching scientific education, making complex concepts more relatable, empowering individuals to envision informed decisions and preventive actions by revisiting the real-world impact of healthcare advancements.
ii. Honing critical thinking to assess traditional pseudoscientific perceptions.
iii. Normalizing the different kinds of emotional comfort that scientific understanding can offer in the larger context. It would lead to a philosophical engagement to fathom existence and purpose from a scientific angle.
iv. Scientifically enhanced cultural understanding by realizing culture as a phenomenon constantly informed and shaped by technological changes in various historical epochs. This shift would enable individuals to exhibit a sense of global connection and navigate technological resistance more clearly and convincingly.
v. Demonstrating the impact of cognitive biases, coping mechanisms, and pattern-seeking behavior on individuals' thought processes and decision-making. It is vital to expose the significance of cognitive biases when encountering psychological biases. It should be followed with conscious habit formation activities to embrace scientific temper in order to decipher scientific explanations and solutions unconsciously.

10.8 CONCLUSION

Integrating IoMT into medical processes offers opportunities and challenges while perceiving the convergence of technology, spirituality, and medical ethics. A posthumanist reading of IoMT developments portrays unparalleled scope for enriching health outcomes and democratizing healthcare accessibility, as well as contesting traditional perceptions of human identity and agency in healthcare. In the future, it is significant to nurture an ecosystem where diverse belief systems do not deter scientific pursuits. It includes continuous interactive dialogue among healthcare providers, ethicists, progressive social activists, believers (the larger populace), and policymakers.

It is essential to drive home the reality that faith healers will not take chances to grow an amputated limb. In contrast, they make tall claims concerning healing conditions that are invisible to the human eye, such as cancer. For instance, following a wrong diagnosis of a malignant tumor, a patient relies on a faith healer. Later, through an effective diagnosis, the patient understands that it is not malignant and attributes healing to the faith healer. However, in the case of amputated limbs, more often than not, rationality prevails even among believers and faith healers, as they do not take chances in trying to pray for growing a limb. Instead, they convince and comfort the patient by stating that it is god's will and that one should be grateful that it is only the limb that is lost and not the life. On the contrary, in such cases, science does not provide such ever-fixated answers; instead, it offers solutions like prosthetic limbs, transplantation surgeries, and IoMT-powered control over prosthetic limbs in the contemporary context.

Such witty yet thought-provoking counternarratives to superstitious grand narratives that offer rationale discourses are imperative to ensure that IoMT developments are effectuated by sensitizing diverse people groups to embrace scientific solutions to improve global healthcare outcomes. Therefore, the future of healthcare lies in this delicate balance— espousing the transformative potential of IoMT and normalizing it among people amidst cultural and spiritual coercion. It is possible by promoting scientific literacy, ensuring democratized accessibility to technology, and nurturing progressive open dialogue between scientific reason and spiritual emotion. Similar initiatives can play a vital role in harnessing the complete potential of IoMT to envision and realize a healthier and inclusive world.

To conclude, posthumanist exploration infers IoMT advancements not just as a technological revolution but also as a philosophical one—reinforcing the perception of what it means to be human in the age of smart, AI-driven, interconnected healthcare devices. As anthropocentric views are continuously challenged by blurring the boundaries between humans and machines in healthcare, remaining vigilant in ethical considerations is crucial to envisioning a health-conscious society. In addition, an empathetic commitment toward equitable access to these sophisticated technologies is also a vital cog. The posthumanist reading reinstates that the future of healthcare may not only rely on the strength of the bodies or the efficiency and expertise of the doctors, but also will depend on the ability to endorse and ethically maneuver the ever-evolving symbiotic relationship between humans and technology. It is apt to end this discourse by stating that in this brave new world of healthcare, humans have already become cyborgs, and that must be the healthiest thing for humanity—indeed, a "speciesist" posthuman perception.

REFERENCES

Ahmed, Haseeb, and Hung Manh La. "Evaluating the Co-Dependence and Co-Existence between Religion and Robots: Past, Present and Insights on the Future." *International Journal of Social Robotics* 13, no. 2 (2021): 219–235.

Akilan, T., U. Hariharan, Immanni Bhanu Prakash, and K. Rajkumar. "Exploring the Impact and Potential of the Internet of Medical Things (IoMT): A Comprehensive Review." In *Proceedings of the 2023 5th International Conference on Advances in Computing, Communication Control and Networking (ICAC3N)*, 967–972. IEEE, 2023.

Al-Turjman, Fadi, Muhammad Haris Nawaz, and Utku Deniz Ulusar. "Intelligence in the Internet of Medical Things Era: A Systematic Review of Current and Future Trends." *Computer Communications* 150 (2020): 644–660.

Alshorman, Omar, Bayan Alshorman, Mahmoud Al-khassaweneh, and Feras Alkahtani. "A Review of Internet of Medical Things (IoMT)-Based Remote Health Monitoring through Wearable Sensors: A Case Study for Diabetic Patients." *Indonesian Journal of Electrical Engineering and Computer Science* 20 (2020): 414–422. https://doi.org/10.11591/IJEECS.V20.I1.PP414-422.

Bakošová, Pavlína, and Juraj Odorčák. "Posthumanism and Human Extinction: Apocalypse, Species, and Two Posthuman Ecologies." *Journal for the Study of Religions and Ideologies* 19, no. 57 (2020): 47–62.

Braidotti, Rosi. *The Posthuman*. Cambridge: Polity Press, 2013.

Buran, Sümeyra, Çağdaş Dedeoğlu, Pınar Kümbet, and Yunus Tuncel. "Posthumanisms beyond Disciplines." *Journal of Posthumanism* 1, no. 1 (2021): 1–4.

Devlin, Mathew. "Cultivating Better Brains: Transhumanism and Its Critics on the Ethics of Enhancement via Brain-Computer Interfacing." Master's thesis, University of Western Ontario, 2014. https://ir.lib.uwo.ca/cgi/viewcontent.cgi?article=3465&context=etd.

Doyle, Darrick. "Pastor: Microchipping Humans Is Straight Out of Revelation." *CBN*, 2017. https://www2.cbn.com/news/us/pastor-microchipping-humans-straight-out-revelation.

Fahmy, Dalia. "Highly Religious Americans More Sceptical of Human Enhancements Such as Brain Implants, Gene Editing." *Pew Research Center*, 2022. https://www.pewresearch.org/short-reads/2022/05/04/highly-religious-americans-more-skeptical-of-human-enhancements-such-as-brain-implants-gene-editing/.

Fiani, Brian, Taylor Reardon, Benjamin Ayres, David Cline, and Sarah R. Sitto. "An Examination of Prospective Uses and Future Directions of Neuralink: The Brain-Machine Interface." *Cureus* 13, no. 3 (2021). https://doi.org/10.7759/cureus.14192.

Foucault, Michel. *The History of Sexuality: Volume 1. The Will to Knowledge*. London: Penguin Classics, 1978.

Foucault, Michel. *Security, Territory, Population: Lectures at the Collège de France, 1977–78*. New York: Springer, 2007.

Ghubaish, Ali, Tarek Salman, Maede Zolanvari, Devrim Unal, Abdulla Al-Ali, and Raj Jain. "Recent Advances in the Internet-of-Medical-Things (IoMT) Systems Security." *IEEE Internet of Things Journal* 8, no. 1 (2020): 8707–8718.

Haraway, Donna. *Simians, Cyborgs, and Women: The Reinvention of Nature*. New York: Routledge, 1991.

Hayles, N. Katherine. *How We Became Posthuman: Virtual Bodies in Cybernetics, Literature, and Informatics*. Chicago: University of Chicago Press, 1999.

Hegde, Satyanarayanan, and Nemr S. Eid. "Telehealth and Remote Patient Monitoring After the COVID Pandemic." *Paediatric Allergy, Immunology, and Pulmonology* 34, no. 4 (2021). https://doi.org/10.1089/ped.2021.0162.

Huang, Chenxi, Jian Wang, Shuihua Wang, and Yudong Zhang. "Internet of Medical Things: A Systematic Review." *Neurocomputing* 557, no. 3 (2023).

Joyia, Gulraiz J., Rao M. Liaqat, Aftab Farooq, and Saad Rehman. "Internet of Medical Things (IoMT): Applications, Benefits and Future Challenges in Healthcare Domain." *Journal of Communications* 12, no. 4 (2017): 240–247.

Khan, Muhammad Farukh, Taser M. Ghazal, Raed A. Said, Areej Fatima, Sagheer Abbas, M.A. Khan, Ghassan F. Issa, Munir Ahmad, and Muhammad Adnan Khan. "An IoMT-Enabled Smart Healthcare Model to Monitor Elderly People Using Machine Learning Technique." *Computational Intelligence and Neuroscience*, 2021.

Krupa, Adam. "Philosophical Concept of Human on the Basis of Posthumanism." *Analiza i Egzystencja* 56 (2021): 75–94.

Latour, Bruno. *Reassembling the Social: An Introduction to Actor-Network-Theory*. Oxford: Oxford University Press, 2005.

Majeed, Fahad, Maria Nazir, and Jens Schneider. "ISA: Internet of Medical Things (IoMT) in Smart Healthcare and Its Applications: A Review." In *Proceedings of the 2023 3rd International Conference on Artificial Intelligence (ICAI)*, 129–135. 2023.

Rashed, Abdelrahman, Ahmed Ibrahim, Ahmed Adel, Bishoy Mourad, Ayman Hatem, Mostafa Magdy, Nada Elgaml, and Ahmed Khattab. "Integrated IoT Medical Platform for Remote Healthcare and Assisted Living." In *2017 Japan-Africa Conference on Electronics, Communications and Computers (JAC-ECC)*, 160–163. 2017. https://doi.org/10.1109/JEC-ECC.2017.8305801.

Razdan, Sahshanu, and Sachin Sharma. "Internet of Medical Things (IoMT): Overview, Emerging Technologies, and Case Studies." *IETE Technical Review* 39, no. 4 (2021): 775–788.

Shakeel, Tanzeela, Shaista Habib, Wadii Boulila, Anis Koubaa, Abdul Rehman Javed, Muhammad Rizwan, Thippa Reddy Gadekallu, and Mahmood Sufiyan. "A Survey on COVID-19 Impact in the Healthcare Domain: Worldwide Market Implementation, Applications, Security and Privacy Issues, Challenges and Future Prospects." *Complex and Intelligent Systems* 9, no. 1 (2023): 1027–1058.

Sharma, Hitesh Kumar, Ravi Tomar, and Preeti. "IoMT and Blockchain-Based Intelligent and Secured System for Smart Healthcare." In *Mathematical Modeling for Intelligent Secured Systems: Theory, Method, and Simulation*, 61–73. CRC Press, 2022.

Srivastava, Jyoti, Sidheswar Routray, Sultan Ahmad, and Mohammad Maqbool Waris. "Internet of Medical Things (IoMT)-Based Smart Healthcare System: Trends and Progress." *Computational Intelligence and Neuroscience*, 2022.

Subha, S., T. M. Inbamalar, Komala C. R., Lakshmi R. Suresh, Sampath Boopathi, and Kamal Alaskar. "A Remote Health Care Monitoring System Using Internet of Medical Things (IoMT)." In *2023 3rd International Conference on Innovative Practices in Technology and Management (ICIPTM)*, 1–6. 2023. https://doi.org/10.1109/ICIPTM57143.2023.10118103.

Subramaniam, Erana Veerappa Dinesh, Kathiravan Srinivasan, Saeed Min Qaisar, and Paweł Pławiak. "Interoperable IoMT Approach for Remote Diagnosis with Privacy-Preservation Perspective in Edge Systems." *Sensors* 23 (2023). https://doi.org/10.3390/s23177474.

Syed, Liyakathunisa, Saima Jabeen, S. Manimala, and Abdullah Alsaeedi. "Smart Healthcare Framework for Ambient Assisted Living Using IoMT and Big Data Analytics Techniques." *Future Generation Computer Systems* (2019). https://doi.org/10.1016/J.FUTURE.2019.06.004.

Toffoletti, Kim. "The Posthuman." *Australian Feminist Studies* 30, no. 85 (2015): 211–213.

Venkatesh, Kavya, Keerthi R, Ikshu B, and Inchara T. Badarish. "Neuralink and Brain Control Machine." *International Journal of Advanced Research in Science, Communication and Technology* (2022): 389–392. https://doi.org/10.48175/ijarsct-3135.

Vilela, Marco, and Leigh R. Hochberg. "Applications of Brain-Computer Interfaces to the Control of Robotic and Prosthetic Arms." In *Handbook of Clinical Neurology*, vol. 168, 87–99. 2020. https://doi.org/10.1016/B978-0-444-63934-9.00008-1.

Vishnu, S. S. R., Jino Ramson, and R. Jegan. "Internet of Medical Things (IoMT) - An Overview." In *2020 5th International Conference on Devices, Circuits and Systems*, 101–104. 2020.

Wong, Shen Yuong, Mian Yu Soh, and Jie Ming Wong. "Internet of Medical Things: Brief Overview and the Future." In *19th IEEE Student Conference on Research and Development: Sustainable Engineering and Technology towards Industry Revolution*, 427–432. 2021.

11 Adverse Childhood Experiences, Psychological Well-Being, and Grit

A Comparative Study between LGBTQIA+ and Cis-Heterogeneous Sample of India

Celina Daniel Satyanadan and Soumya R.R.

11.1 INTRODUCTION

11.1.1 Adverse Childhood Experiences (ACEs)

ACEs are severe and traumatic childhood events in a child's life that comprise of physical, emotional, or sexual abuse; neglect; and household dysfunction, such as witnessing abuse at home or substance addiction (Felitti et al., 1998). As a result, the impacts of ACEs on an individual's overall health are substantial. They are more likely to develop chronic diseases, substance dependence, and behavioral health problems and die at a younger age than their unexposed peers (Rogers et al., 2022; Sonu et al., 2019; Chapman et al., 2004). Furthermore, ACEs have an adverse economic and social impact, reducing educational achievement, work opportunities, and boosting criminal involvement (Felitti et al., 1998). According to a 2022 study published in the journal *Child Abuse & Neglect*, the prevalence of ACEs in Sexual and Gender Minorities (SGM) youth in India is high, with an estimated 86% of SGM youth reporting at least one ACE. The most common types of ACEs reported by SGM youth in India were emotional abuse (58%), physical abuse (48%), and sexual abuse (37%).

DOI: 10.1201/9781003476344-11

11.1.2 Psychological Well-Being (PWB)

PWB is vital for physical health, cognitive functioning, and happiness, which comprise of dimensions such as autonomy, environmental mastery, personal growth, positive relations, purpose in life, and self-acceptance (Ryff & Keyes, 1995). Autonomy is associated with individual decision-making and the orientation toward direction, and its strength as a predictor of well-being also correlates with higher life satisfaction and better mental and physical health (Ryff, 1989; Ryff & Keyes, 1995). Environmental mastery is another significant indicator that depends on controlling one's environment, addressing challenges, and using all available resources, and its strength as a predictor is second only to autonomy (Ryff, 1989; Ryff & Keyes, 1995). Personal growth signifies continuous development, openness to new experiences, and realizing one's potential, making it the third strongest predictor of PWB (Ryff, 1989; Ryff & Keyes, 1995). Forming positive relations with others involves the capacity to establish and preserve fulfilling relationships with people in one's social context. This entails sharing closeness, mutual respect, and trust with others, as well as feeling a sense of belonging and connectedness in relationships (Ryff, 1989). Purpose in life is the feeling that one's life has significance and direction, and that one is making a valuable contribution to the world. On the other hand, self-acceptance includes recognizing one's strengths and weaknesses and having a positive outlook on oneself in life. This also includes one's past experiences, which has been linked to subjective well-being (Ryff, 1989; Su et al., 2019). In psychology, PWB has been widely employed and validated.

11.1.3 Grit

Grit is referred to as a personality trait characterized by perseverance and passion for long-term goals and the ability to maintain effort and persistence over time despite hardship, setbacks, and failures (Duckworth & Quinn, 2009). Grit has also been defined as maintaining focus and motivation toward the same objectives over time (Datu, 2021).

11.2 THEORETICAL FRAMEWORK

11.2.1 The Minority Stress Model

For sexual orientation–based differences in India, one framework to understand the possibilities is the minority stress model by Meyer (2003). The model begins with the premise that social factors, such as discrimination, bias, and oppression, can contribute to the marginalization of groups and result in increased stress and increases in different health conditions. This stress is identified as "minority stress" which is connected to a range of negative health repercussions, including but not restricted to, depressive disorders, anxiety, addiction, and chronic diseases (Meyer, 2003). The model also suggests that SGM can use various coping mechanisms to manage minority stress, including some that are adaptive for them, and some, like substance use, which are dangerous. Thus, it may be assumed that sexual and gender minorities who are victims of harassment will demonstrate more obvious psychological effects due to being comparatively stressed in general (Meyer, 2003).

11.3 CONCEPTUAL FRAMEWORK

While ACEs are prevalent among various populations, sexual and gender minorities (SGM) face a heightened risk. Research indicates that LGBTQIA+ youth have distinct patterns of ACEs, with higher scores in 9 out of 10 ACE categories. Notably, emotional neglect, emotional abuse, and living with a family member with mental illness are common ACEs for gender minorities (Craig et al., 2020). Additionally, studies in India highlight that sexual minorities are more susceptible to physical, sexual, economic, and emotional violence from the general community (Khan et al., 2009). PWB and grit significantly contribute to resilience and coping in adversity. For instance, PWB is linked to resilience in Chinese college students (Huang et al., 2021). Thus, investigating ACEs, PWB, and grit among gender and sexual minorities (SGM) becomes even more crucial.

11.4 NEED AND SIGNIFICANCE

Conducting a comparative study between sexual and gender minorities and cis-heterogeneous people may be very beneficial as well as it can help determine the extent of disparities within SGM compared to the general population. It will help identify specific areas of lower PWB in SGM and develop targeted interventions and resilience-promoting strategies. The research can directly contribute to the work of community organizations, as well as clinical practice, helping organizations develop more targeted services and better assist SGM with history of ACEs. In addition, the findings can be used to raise awareness and educate the broader public about SGM's specific needs and help reduce stigma and discrimination in a country like India.

11.5 REVIEW OF LITERATURE

Several researches have investigated the occurrence and impacts of ACEs in gender and sexual minorities. According to the findings of research in the US gender minorities, ACEs are related to lower physical and mental health outcomes while resilience moderates this relationship. The study discovered that higher levels of resilience were related with improved physical and mental health outcomes, even among people who had encountered a high number of ACEs (Schnarrs et al., 2020).

ACEs also have an impact on substance use behavior in gender minorities (Dowling et al., 2023). Further, a study attempted to investigate the differences in ACEs and quality of physical and mental health between transgender and cisgender sexual minorities. It was found that overall, 51% of the transgender sample had at least four ACEs, compared to 12.6% heterosexual people and 30.5% LGB adults. The findings indicated that childhood neglect was a prevalent event among LGB individuals (Schnarrs et al., 2019).

According to the studies carried out by Schilling et al. (2007), cisgender people with four or more ACEs were at significantly higher risk of mental health problems than those with less ACEs. These also show that more ACEs are associated with increased psychological distress, and a lower general self-efficacy, while a decreased general self-efficacy was related to heightened psychological distress (Belloir et al., 2023). Another research explains that people with at least four categories of childhood exposure to ACEs faced significantly higher chances of suffering from severe issues like alcoholism, drug abuse, depression, and suicide attempts (4–12 times higher), as well as smoking, poor self-rated health, and sexually transmitted diseases (2–4 times higher) among other things. Physical inactivity and serious obesity were also up to 1.6 times more likely in individuals exposed to four or more categories of ACE's during their childhood. The presence of adult diseases such as ischemic heart disease, cancer, and chronic lung disease was related to the number of adverse child exposures experienced (Felitti et al., 1998). Additionally, they were found to be 1.4–1.6 times more likely to experience physical inactivity and severe obesity.

Numerous studies have researched into how childhood experiences impact mental health and overall well-being. One such study found that when factors like age, gender, and socioeconomic status were considered, ACEs were linked to poorer PWB and higher rates of substance use (Hanif et al., 2022).

In terms of ACEs and grit, evidence-based investigations have revealed significant negative effects of ACEs on grit, while mindfulness was found to have a positive impact on grit. This suggests that mindfulness plays a crucial mediating role in the ACEs–grit relationship, indicating the potential for mindfulness-based therapies to enhance grit, especially in at-risk populations (Cheung et al., 2022). Another study identified gender disparities in resilience and the influence of experiences like physical abuse, physical fighting, and indirect communal violence. The relationship between ACEs and resilience was mediated by gender, with female individuals reporting a higher prevalence of ACEs (Pasha-Zaidi et al., 2020).

Grit and ACEs have been linked in previous studies. For example, in a study of Chinese college students, ACEs, particularly abuse and neglect, significantly affected grit (Cheung et al., 2022).

Moreover, PWB is also associated with grit. Research on nursing students found that academic resilience, grit, and satisfaction were significant predictors of PWB (Jin & Kim, 2017). However, little research has explored the relationship between grit and PWB in gender minorities. Studies have also shown that resilience and grit are linked to PWB (Vinothkumar & Prasad, 2016), and grit can reduce burnout and enhance PWB, as seen in medical students (Shih & Maroongroge, 2017). PWB in gender minorities has been studied globally. Lower levels of PWB are associated with gender non-conformity, and perceived experiences of stigmatization mediate this relationship (Baams et al., 2013).

11.6 RESEARCH PROBLEM

Growing up in difficult circumstances or having adverse and traumatic childhood experiences can affect how people feel about themselves and how they manage later in life. It can affect both the physical and mental health of such people, and it can also make it harder to connect with others, especially for people who identify as sexual or gender minorities (SGM). Because SGM individuals often face more challenges in their lives and struggle with mental health more than others, they are particularly at risk when it comes to these kinds of difficulties. Hence it is important to find out if LGBTQIA+ individuals experience these situations more often than those who identify as heterosexual.

11.7 METHOD

11.7.1 Aim

To understand the variations in ACEs, PWB, and grit between sexual and gender minorities (SGM) and a cis-heterogeneous sample of individuals aged between 18 and 25 in India.

11.7.2 HYPOTHESIS

$H_0$1: There are no significant differences in the ACEs scores of cis-heterogeneous sample and LGBTQIA+ sample of India.
$H_0$2: There are no significant differences in the grit scores of cis-heterogeneous sample and LGBTQIA+ sample of India.
$H_0$3: There are no significant differences in the dimension scores of PWB between cis-heterogeneous sample and LGBTQIA+ sample of India.

11.7.3 RESEARCH DESIGN

This study employed a cross-sectional, comparative design to investigate variations in ACEs, PWB, and grit among a sample of India's LGBTQIA+ community and a sample representing cisgender individuals with diverse backgrounds.

11.7.4 OPERATIONAL DEFINITIONS

11.7.4.1 Independent Variables

Sexual orientation and gender identity: In this study, participants were first asked to tick their gender and sexual orientation according to what they identify as. Later, they were split into two groups based on their answers: one group included people who feel their gender matches the one they were assigned at birth, called the cis-heterogeneous group. The other group consisted of people who see themselves as part of the LGBTQIA+ community, which covers lesbian, gay, bisexual, transgender, queer, intersex, asexual, or questioning individuals. This group was referred to as the sexual and gender minority (SGM) category.

11.7.4.2 Dependent Variables

Adverse childhood experiences: In this study, the ACE questionnaire was used to operationalize childhood experiences that were traumatic. This questionnaire asked participants about ten different things related to abuse, neglect, and family issues that might have happened during their childhood. Higher scores on this questionnaire indicated a greater number of ACEs.

Grit: In the current study, grit was operationalized as a score on the Grit Scale which ranges from 1 to 5. Higher grit scores indicate greater grit and lower scores indicate lower grit.

Psychological well-being: Scores on the Ryff's psychological well-being scale was used to operationalize PWB. Higher scores indicate greater PWB as compared to low scores on the scale.

11.7.5 SAMPLE

A total sample size of 220 was drawn from both the populations, with 102 samples drawn from SGM and 118 from cis-heterogeneous populations. Convenience sampling was opted to gather data, as it is a method commonly used when it is challenging to access a representative sample, particularly for minority populations like SGM.

11.7.5.1 Inclusion Criteria

The SGM sample included individuals aged between 18 and 25 who identified as LGBTQIA+ and other diverse gender and sexual identities. The cis-heterogeneous sample consisted of individuals aged between 18 and 25 whose gender identity aligned with their assigned sex at birth and who were attracted to people of the opposite gender. The chosen age range was essential for assessing ACEs up to age 17 and for understanding how early life experiences may influence the formation of personal and gender identity during this critical period.

11.7.5.2 Exclusion Criteria

The exclusion criteria included individuals who reside outside India and who are diagnosed with a mental disorder in both the populations.

11.7.6 TOOLS

Adverse childhood experiences: In order to measure the levels of ACEs, the ACEs questionnaire was used. It consists of ten items that assess different types of childhood trauma, including physical, sexual, and emotional abuse, neglect, and household dysfunction. The psychometric properties of this questionnaire have been thoroughly investigated. The ACE questionnaire has a test–retest reliability between

0.60 and 0.87. Dube et al. (2003) reported a Cronbach's alpha of 0.81 (Dube et al., 2003).

Psychological well-being: PWB was measured using Ryff's scale of PWB which is a 42-item scale. Six dimensions of PWB are measured by this scale:

1. *Autonomy:* An individual's sense of self-determination, independence, and mastery over their lives.
2. *Environmental mastery:* The degree to which individuals believe they are competent and effective in managing their surroundings and attaining their objectives.
3. *Personal growth:* An individual's sense of ongoing growth and development, as well as their drive to learn and explore new things.
4. *Positive relations with others:* The amount to which individuals experience gratifying and meaningful interpersonal relationships and feel connected to their community.
5. *Purpose in life:* The degree to which individuals believe they have a feeling of purpose and meaning in their lives, and that their activities are meaningful and significant.
6. *Self-acceptance:* The degree to which people have favorable feelings about themselves and accept themselves for who they are, including their flaws.

The RPWB has good internal consistency for each subscale, with Cronbach's alpha coefficients ranging from .76 to .88 (Ryff & Keyes, 1995).

Grit: Grit was measured using the Grit Scale, developed by psychologist Angela Duckworth. It is a self-report measure of perseverance and passion for long-term goals. It consists of 12 items that evaluate two aspects of grit: persistence in effort and consistency of interest. The Grit Scale has strong internal consistency, with Cronbach's alpha coefficients ranging from .70 to .90 across different samples (Duckworth et al., 2007; Eskreis-Winkler et al., 2016; Credé et al., 2017). Grit also has good internal consistency (Cronbach's alpha = .82) and test–retest reliability (r = .83), and was positively correlated with academic achievement and conscientiousness in Indian undergraduates. It also has good predictive validity for factors such as academic achievement, employment performance and athletic performance, IQ, and personality (Duckworth et al., 2007; Eskreis-Winkler et al., 2016; Credé et al., 2017).

11.7.7 PROCEDURE

The study gathered 220 individuals, with 118 from the cisgender heterogeneous group and 102 from the sexual and gender minority (SGM) group. The researchers used various recruitment methods, including in-person interactions, online forums, social media platforms, and community organizations to ensure a broad and diverse participant pool. Before proceeding with the questionnaires, participants were provided with detailed instructions about the study's purpose, time commitment, and other relevant information. They were also given the opportunity to seek clarification or ask questions before beginning the questionnaire.

11.7.8 DATA ANALYSIS

Post the completion of data collection, descriptive statistics, i.e., mean, median, and standard deviations for all the three variables of ACEs, grit, and PWB were computed using the software Jamovi. Finally, an independent sample *t*-test was run on Statistical Package for Social Sciences (SPSS) 2.0 version, between the two groups to compare significant differences in these variables between the cis heterogeneous and gender and sexual minorities (SGM) sample.

11.7.9 ETHICAL CONSIDERATIONS

Ethical considerations were maintained throughout the research, i.e., the sample were asked for informed consent before participating and were made aware of their right to withdraw from the study at any given time without explanation. The confidentiality and privacy of the data provided by the sample were kept anonymous and were only accessible by the researcher and their supervisor. A precautionary step was taken by the researcher to reduce the risk of harm by referring resources for support or mental health experts to the participants if necessary. The researcher strived to be inclusive and respectful of the sample's different identities, experiences, and perspectives throughout the research.

11.8 RESULTS

11.8.1 Descriptive Statistics

In Table 11.1, the average age of respondents is 21 (SD = 1.94). Furthermore, the youngest response is 18 years old, while the oldest is 25 years old.

In Table 11.2, the mean value of ACEs score is 1.17 (SD = 1.65). Additionally, the lowest score is 0 and highest score is 7. Similarly, the mean value of Grit scores is 2.69 (SD = 0.41). Furthermore, the lowest score is 1.58 and highest score is 3.92.

In Table 11.3, the mean value of autonomy, environmental mastery, personal growth, personal relations with others, purpose in life, and self-acceptance scores are 31.2, 29.3, 35.5, 34.2, 32.3, and 30.4, respectively. Similarly, the standard deviations for the same are 6.41, 6.17, 6.69, 6.0, 6.59, and 7.12, respectively. As can be seen, individuals have the highest mean score in personal growth and lowest in environmental mastery.

TABLE 11.1
Age (Cis-Heterogeneous Sample)

	N	*M*	Median	Std. Dev.	Min	Max
Age	118	21	21	1.94	18	25

TABLE 11.2
Adverse Childhood Experiences (ACE) and Grit of Cis-Heterogeneous Sample

	N	*M*	Median	Std. Dev.	Min	Max
ACE	118	1.17	1	1.65	0.0	7.0
Grit	118	2.69	2.67	0.417	1.58	3.92

TABLE 11.3
Psychological Well-Being of Cis-Heterogeneous Sample

	N	*M*	Median	Std. Dev	,Min	Max
Autonomy	118	31.2	30.0	6.41	12	49
Environmental mastery	118	29.3	29.0	6.17	15	43
Personal growth	118	35.5	36.0	6.69	19	49
Positive relations with others	118	34.2	34.0	6.0	12	49
Purpose in life	118	32.3	31.5	6.59	16	48
Self-acceptance	118	30.4	30.0	7.12	11	49

Table 11.4 shows the average age of respondents in LGBTQIA+ sample as 20.4 (SD = 2.13). Furthermore, the youngest response is 18 years old, while the oldest is 25 years old.

Table 11.5 shows the mean value of ACEs scores in the LGBTQIA+ sample as 3.02 (SD = 2.08). Additionally, the lowest score is 0 and the highest score is 9. Similarly, the mean value of grit scores is 2.56 (SD = 0.45). Furthermore, the lowest score is 1 and highest score is 3.42.

Table 11.6 shows the mean value of autonomy, environmental mastery, personal growth, personal relations with others, purpose in life, and self-acceptance scores as 29.5, 24, 34.4, 31.8, 31.2, and 24.9, respectively. Similarly, the standard deviations for the same are 7.97, 6.82, 6.51, 8.19, 8.21, and 6.87, respectively. As can be seen, individuals have the highest mean score in personal growth and lowest in self-acceptance.

TABLE 11.4
Age (LGBTQIA+ Sample)

	N	*M*	Median	Std. Dev.	Min	Max
Age	102	20.4	20.0	2.13	18	25

TABLE 11.5
Adverse Childhood Experiences (ACE) and Grit of LGBTQIA+ Sample

	N	*M*	Median	Std. Dev.	Min	Max
ACE	102	3.02	3.0	2.08	0.0	9.0
Grit	102	2.56	2.58	0.445	1.0	3.42

TABLE 11.6
Psychological Well-Being of LGBTQIA+ Sample

	N	*M*	Median	Std. Dev.	Min	Max
Autonomy	102	29.5	29.0	7.97	10	49
Environmental mastery	102	24.0	24.0	6.82	10	40
Personal growth	102	34.4	34.0	6.51	20	49
Positive relations with others	102	31.8	32.0	8.19	15	49
Purpose in life	102	31.2	31.0	8.21	14	48
Self-acceptance	102	24.9	25.5	6.87	8	40

11.8.2 Inferential Statistics

An independent sample *t*-test was conducted to compare the differences between the variables of ACEs, grit, and the dimensions of PWB among the cis-heterogeneous and LGBTQIA+ sample. In this study, independent samples *t*-test is an appropriate measure as the aim is to investigate potential differences in ACEs, grit, and PWB between these two independent groups of cis-heterogeneous and sexual and gender minority samples.

In Table 11.7, there were significant differences (t (191.9) = –7.267, p <.001) between the two groups in terms of ACEs where mean score for LGBTQIA+ sample (M = 3.02, SD = 2.08) was higher than the cis-heterogeneous sample (M = 1.17, SD = 1.65). Hence, we reject the null hypothesis that states that there are no significant differences in the ACEs of cis-heterogeneous and LGBTQIA+ sample. Further, there were significant differences (t (218) = 2.255, p <.05) between the two groups in their grit where the mean value of cis-heterogeneous sample (M = 2.69, SD = 0.417) was higher than the LGBTQIA+ sample (M = 2.56, SD = 0.445. Hence, we reject the null hypothesis that states that there are no significant differences in the grit scores of cis-heterogeneous and LGBTQIA+ sample.

Under PWB, there were no significant differences (t (193.4) = 1.749, p >.05) between the two groups in the context of autonomy. Furthermore, there were also no significant differences between the two groups in the context of purpose in life (t (193.22) = 1.038, p >.05). Also, no significant differences were found in the dimension of personal growth (t (218) = 1.176, p >.05).

TABLE 11.7
Independent Samples *t*-Test for ACE, Grit, and PWB

	Homogeneity of Variance	Levene's Test for Equality of Variances	*t*	*df*	Sig (2 tailed)
ACE	Equal variances not assumed	0.01	−7.267	191.9	.000***
Grit	Equal variances assumed	.874	2.255	218	.025*
Autonomy	Equal variances not assumed	.025	1.749	193.4	.082
Environmental mastery	Equal variances assumed	.241	5.953	218	.000***
Personal growth	Equal variances assumed	.556	1.176	218	.241
Positive relation with others	Equal variances not assumed	.001	2.539	182.40005	.012*
Purpose in life	Equal variances not assumed	.022	1.038	193.22	.300
Self-acceptance	Equal variances assumed	.732	5.860	218	.000***

Note: $p < 0.05$*, $p < 0.001$***.

However, there were significant differences in the dimension of positive relations with others (t (182.40) = 2.539, p <.05) where the mean score for the LGBTQIA+ sample (M = 31.8, SD = 8.19) was lower than the cis-heterogeneous sample (M = 34.2, SD = 6.0). Also, there were significant differences in Environmental Mastery (t (218) = 5.953, p <.001) where mean score for LGBTQIA+ sample (M = 24. SD = 6.82) was lower than the cis-heterogeneous sample (M = 29.3, SD = 6.17). Moreover, there were significant differences in self-acceptance (t (218) = 5.860, p < .001) between the cis-heterogeneous and LGBTQIA+ sample where the mean score for LGBTQIA+ sample (M = 24.9, SD = 6.87) was lower than the cis-heterogeneous sample (M = 30.4, SD = 7.1)

Since there is a difference between three dimensions of PWB, we reject the null hypothesis that states that there are no significant differences in the dimension scores of PWB of cis-heterogeneous and LGBTQIA+ sample.

11.9 DISCUSSION

This study compared ACE, PWB, and grit in the LGBTQIA+ and cis-heterogeneous populations in India. Findings indicate significant differences between the two groups in this aspect. Moreover, descriptive statistics indicate higher ACEs in the LGBTQIA+ sample. Prior research supports these results. For instance, LGBTQIA+ youth show distinct ACE patterns, scoring higher in nine out of ten categories, with common ACEs including emotional neglect (58%) and abuse (56%) (Craig et al., 2020). Another study by McCabe et al. (2020) explored ACEs in sexual orientation subgroups. Bisexual women had the highest ACE frequency and co-occurring substance use and mental health issues, with 43.8% reporting four or more ACEs. Sexual minorities consistently had higher ACE means, often with co-occurring mental health and substance use problems.

A different research study investigated the occurrence of childhood physical, emotional, and sexual abuse, as well as childhood household dysfunction, among both sexual minority and heterosexual adults. The findings indicated that when compared to heterosexual participants, gay/lesbian individuals showed elevated odds for six out of eight ACEs, while bisexual individuals exhibited increased odds for seven out of eight such experiences (Andersen & Blosnich, 2013). Another study also revealed that transgender individuals reported more emotional abuse, physical neglect, and emotional neglect than cisgender LGB people and the findings also demonstrated that neglect is a common experience among the sexual and gender minority people and that it should be evaluated with other ACE categories (Schnarrs et al., 2019).

It is rather common for LGBTQIA+ children to experience bullying and victimization in school settings, as noted by Kosciw et al. (2016). This mistreatment often leads to psychological scars and adds to their ACEs. Because of these challenges, LGBTQIA+ individuals often struggle with mental health issues like depression and anxiety, as highlighted by the Institute of Medicine in 2011. These mental health disparities can both stem from and worsen the adverse experiences they face.

In this study, it was found that among the categories of ACEs, the LGBTQIA+ participants reported the highest levels of psychological, sexual, and physical abuse.

Friedman et al. (2011) conducted a meta-analysis indicating that children and teenagers who undergo sexual abuse are at a heightened risk of encountering various mental health and behavioral challenges, including depression, posttraumatic stress disorder, and substance abuse disorders. Moreover, observing parental physical abuse is associated with psychological issues, substance abuse, behavioral problems, and involvement in criminal activities (Friedman et al., 2011). Furthermore, sexual minority youth are more likely to endure sexual abuse, parental physical abuse, and peer victimization during childhood compared to their heterosexual counterparts (Friedman et al., 2011).

This study also aimed to assess grit in LGBTQIA+ and cis-heterogeneous groups, finding significant differences between them and descriptive statistics showing lower grit mean for the SGM sample. Constant stress and marginalization can negatively impact mental health and well-being, leading to lower levels of resilience and perseverance, key components of grit in the LGBTQIA+ sample. A study found that gay men ageing with HIV in regional Queensland demonstrated significant grit in overcoming challenges. This resilience was attributed to strong social support networks, positive self-identity, embracing their identities, and finding meaning and purpose in life helped these men overcome societal negativity and discrimination (Gardiner, 2018). Since these aspects are often found in lower levels in the Indian gender and sexual minorities, these factors help explain the lower mean score of grit in this minority sample.

Another potential factor contributing to lower levels of grit in the SGM sample could be internalized homophobia. For example, research has explored how gay and bisexual men cope with negative feelings about their sexuality (internalized homophobia) over time and its impact on their health. The findings revealed that many men were able to overcome these feelings over time, irrespective of factors such as age, race, or education level. Those who successfully tackled internalized homophobia tended to experience better overall health compared to those who did not. These results highlight the resilience exhibited by participants, which is associated with positive health outcomes (Herrick et al., 2013). Therefore, the presence of higher levels of internalized homophobia may help elucidate the lower levels of grit observed in this population.

Nevertheless, studies have aimed at studying strategies that can help sexual and gender minorities to enhance resilience. For instance, Russell and Richards (2003) studied the stresses and factors that lead to resilience for gay and bisexual males in Colorado following the passage of anti-gay laws that denied them legal recourse for sexual orientation discrimination. This study identified five sources of resiliency in LGB individuals through anti-gay behavior: (1) the capacity to turn anti-LGBTQ politics from a negative to a positive social movement; (2) facing down internalized homophobia; (3) expressing emotions (like anger or sadness); (4) effective witnessing and receiving support from others (especially from the heterosexual community); and (5) greater support from the LGBT community (Russell & Richards, 2003). Additionally, access to LGBTQIA+ affirming mental health services and resources can contribute to the grit of sexual and gender minority individuals. For instance, a study showed that mindfulness-based cognitive therapy increased grit levels in a university sample (Rusadi et al., 2021).

Furthermore, in terms of PWB, there were significant differences between LGBTQIA+ and cis-heterogeneous sample in terms of environmental mastery, positive relations with others, and self-acceptance. From a closer look, it is evident that sexual and gender minorities have lower scores in these respective domains.

The LGBTQIA+ group's low scores and struggles with environmental mastery suggest they face difficulties in shaping their surroundings to match their needs and desires. This could be due to a range of factors, including discrimination and prejudice. LGBTQIA+ individuals often encounter societal discrimination and prejudice, which can make it harder for them to access resources, opportunities, and supportive environments (Meyer, 2003). Additionally, dealing with minority stress which is constantly facing stressors tied to being a minority, like microaggressions and invalidation, can drain their energy and make it difficult to navigate and impact their surroundings (Meyer, 2003). Furthermore, internalized stigma, i.e., absorbing negative social attitudes toward LGBTQIA+ identities can affect their confidence and make them doubt their ability to shape their environment (Herek, 2009).

Furthermore, LGBTQIA+ people are more likely to be victimized and bullied, both as adolescents and adults. These experiences can lead to a lower sense of safety, increased stress levels, and diminished confidence in efficiently regulating their environment (Fish et al., 2023). Moreover, environmental mastery may also be impacted by the constitutional and legal framework regarding LGBTQIA+ rights. LGBTQIA+ people may encounter significant obstacles when trying to access opportunities, resources, and supportive settings in places with inadequate legal protections or discriminatory laws (Richman & Hatzenbuehler, 2014). LGBTQIA+ people, for instance, are still not allowed to marry in India, which makes it more difficult for them to alter their environment to suit their requirements and preferences.

In addition, the lower scores in positive relations with others in the LGBTQIA+ group might be linked to experiences of social isolation, rejection, and stigma. Social support is crucial for PWB, and its absence can negatively impact mental health and well-being (Thoits, 2011). This has been the case in the present study as well. Factors contributing to this include family rejection i.e., lack of familial acceptance and support can be particularly detrimental to LGBTQIA+ individuals, leading to feelings of isolation and loneliness (Eres et al., 2021). Another factor is heteronormativity. For instance, a study showed that nurses may believe that all patients are heterosexual, and these heteronormative assumptions can lead to poor communication, lowering nursing quality by causing nurses to ask inappropriate questions and make erroneous judgements (Röndahl et al., 2006). Hence, this shows that societal expectations and assumptions about heterosexuality can create barriers to forming meaningful relationships for LGBTQIA+ individuals. Along with this, fear of discrimination or anticipation of discrimination and prejudice can limit engagement with others and hinder the development of strong social bonds (Juda, 2021).

Also, the lower self-acceptance scores in the LGBTQIA+ group highlight the challenges many face in internalizing and affirming their identities. Apart from the above-mentioned reasons, LGBTQIA+ individuals' self-acceptance might be influenced by their cultural and religious views. Some cultural or religious contexts may have conservative or non-affirming attitudes toward sexual orientation or gender identity, which can present further barriers to self-acceptance (Lefevor et al., 2020). Moreover, comparing themselves to their peers or to social media figures can lead to lower self-acceptance. For instance, a study found individuals often compare themselves to the way influencers present themselves online and see them as representing an ideal version of themselves. This comparison can lead to feelings of both dissatisfaction and low self-acceptance (Shehzala et al., 2024).

Researchers found in a recent study that there was a correlation between experiencing greater pressures related to being a sexual minority and feeling less accepting of one's sexuality. These pressures included coping with internalized beliefs that support heterosexuality, keeping one's identity a secret, and dealing with rejection from friends and family (Camp et al., 2020). Moreover, lack of positive role models and limited exposure to positive and affirming representations of LGBTQIA+ individuals can make it difficult to develop a strong sense of self-acceptance. For example, in a study, participants from various ethnic backgrounds highlighted how their adolescence experiences with and without role models influenced their queer identification as a Black and Indigenous Persons of Color (BIPOC) lesbian female. Results suggest that having a BIPOC lesbian female, cisgender, or transgender role model in popular media can empower young people to come out and develop their queer identity during adolescence. Role models inspired LGBT adolescents to seek achievement and positive outcomes similar to those they admired (Gomillion & Giuliano, 2011).

In conclusion, promoting PWB in gender and sexual minorities is vital due to their unique challenges. Research suggests key strategies: providing culturally competent mental health services (Bockting et al., 2013), fostering supportive social networks (Frost et al., 2013), advocating anti-discrimination policies (Hatzenbuehler, 2010), and ensuring access to LGBTQ+-affirming mental health professionals (Meyer, 2003). Research has demonstrated that participating in interventions that validate LGBTQ+ identities, obtaining knowledge, and being a part of a supportive community can enhance one's general well-being (Rosario et al., 1996; Herek et al., 2009; Busseri et al., 2006).

11.10 SUMMARY OF FINDINGS

This study found substantial variations in unfavorable childhood experiences between the cisgender heterosexual and LGBTQIA+ populations. There were also noticeable differences in the two groups' grit levels. Likewise, noteworthy distinctions were noted among PWB in terms of environmental mastery, positive interpersonal relationships, and self-acceptance.

11.11 IMPLICATIONS

This research has substantial implications that can be noted. First, the significant differences in ACEs between the LGBTQIA+ and cis-heterogeneous samples highlight the need for tailored mental health interventions for the sexual and gender minorities. Initiatives aimed at addressing and mitigating the impact of ACEs should be developed, with a focus on LGBTQIA+ individuals who may be at higher risk. Further, lower levels of environmental mastery, positive relations with others, and self-acceptance in the LGBTQIA+ sample highlight the importance of psychosocial interventions such as group therapy and family therapy which can be helpful to increase these categories of PWB.

These findings of this research can be used to support mental health policies that recognize and address the unique challenges and strengths of LGBTQIA+ individuals. There is also little access to licensed guidance counsellors, gender-neutral restrooms, LGBT literature, and non-heteronormative sex education in India and hence, this research is aimed at increasing advocacy in these aspects and reducing disparities and promoting equitable access to mental health resources in this minority sample. The study emphasizes the importance of culturally competent mental health services and support within the context of India. This includes ensuring that mental health professionals are trained to work effectively with people from diverse sexual orientations and gender identities. The research can inform educational programs and awareness campaigns focused on promoting mental health and well-being. These activities have the potential to reduce stigma and raise awareness of the mental health challenges that many groups in the community face, particularly in India.

11.12 LIMITATIONS

The study's findings may not accurately reflect the complete LGBTQIA+ and cis-heterogeneous groups in India. Those that volunteered for the study may have different characteristics than those who did not, resulting in a biased sample. Furthermore, some participants may have been hesitant to share their LGBTQIA+ identification or experiences for fear of stigma or prejudice, causing them to withhold essential information. Furthermore, the information gathered about ACEs and mental health is based on people's memories and honesty, which might be influenced by biases or a desire to look a specific way. People may not remember or report information accurately. This might have led to recall bias or social desirability bias. Additionally, the study did not take into account other factors that could influence mental well-being and grit, such as socioeconomic status, availability of mental health services, or the level of support from one's community.

11.13 SCOPE FOR FUTURE RESEARCH

While this study has provided valuable insights, further research is needed to explore the specific factors contributing to differences in ACEs in the SGM group. Qualitative investigations can offer deeper insights into the experiences and needs of LGBTQIA+ individuals. For instance, future researchers can conduct qualitative studies to explore the unique struggles that minority individuals have faced in their childhood that have contributed to their adverse experiences. In addition, building on the initial comparative study, conducting a long-term longitudinal study could provide insights into the changes in PWB and grit over time within both LGBTQIA+ and cis-heterogeneous populations. Understanding these data could help identify critical stages of development and create effective therapies. Future studies can also investigate how cultural and geographical differences in India influence the relationships between ACEs, PWB, and grit. Given India's great cultural diversity, recognizing regional variances is critical for a complete understanding. Additionally, future researchers can explore the intersectionality of identity factors, such as gender, caste, socioeconomic status, and disability, within the LGBTQIA+ and cis-heterogeneous populations and how these factors interact with ACEs to influence well-being.

11.14 CONCLUSION

In conclusion, this study paints a distressing image of the LGBTQIA+ community in India, indicating a group that struggles with poorer levels of resilience, grit, and well-being than their cisgender heterosexual peers, as well as greater rates of ACEs. These findings highlight the need for a comprehensive approach to addressing these inequities. It is critical to prioritize culturally sensitive mental health services that are customized to the unique needs of LGBTQIA+ people. Furthermore, creating safe spaces and encouraging social relationships in the community can provide crucial support and a sense of belonging. Additionally, addressing prejudice and societal stigma through legal reforms or educational programs is critical to building a more inclusive workplace. Finally, increasing understanding and acceptance within families can have a substantial impact on the well-being of LGBTQIA+ people. By actively promoting inclusion in all aspects of society, we can create a more accepting and uplifting environment in which individuals in India can thrive.

REFERENCES

Andersen, J. P., & Blosnich, J. R. (2013). Disparities in adverse childhood experiences among sexual minority and heterosexual adults: Results from a multi-state probability-based sample. *PLoS One*, *8*(1), e54691. https://doi.org/10.1371/journal.pone.0054691

Baams, L., Beek, T. F., Hille, H., Zevenbergen, F., & Bos, H. M. W. (2013). Gender nonconformity, perceived stigmatization, and psychological well-being in Dutch sexual minority youth and young adults: A mediation analysis. *Archives of Sexual Behavior*, *42*(5), 765–773. https://doi.org/10.1007/s10508-012-0055-z

Belloir, J. A., Fabiano, F., Jackman, K. B., & Bockting, W. O. (2023). General self-efficacy as a mediator of the association between adverse childhood experiences and psychological distress in gender-minority individuals. *Journal of Nursing Scholarship*. https://doi.org/10.1111/jnu.12889

Bockting, W., Miner, M. H., Romine, R. E. S., Hamilton, A. R., & Coleman, E. (2013). Stigma, mental health, and resilience in an online sample of the US transgender population. *American Journal of Public Health*, *103*(5), 943–951. https://doi.org/10.2105/ajph.2013.301241

Busseri, M. A., Willoughby, T., Chalmers, H., & Bogaert, A. R. (2006). Same-sex attraction and successful adolescent development. *Journal of Youth and Adolescence*, *35*(4), 561–573. https://doi.org/10.1007/s10964-006-9071-4

Camp, J., Vitoratou, S., & Rimes, K. A. (2020). LGBQ+ self-acceptance and its relationship with minority stressors and mental health: A systematic literature review. *Archives of Sexual Behavior, 49*(7), 2353–2373. https://doi.org/10.1007/s10508-020-01755-2

Chapman, D. P., Whitfield, C. W., Felitti, V. J., Dube, S. R., Edwards, V. J., & Anda, R. F. (2004). Adverse childhood experiences and the risk of depressive disorders in adulthood. *Journal of Affective Disorders, 82*(2), 217–225. https://doi.org/10.1016/j.jad.2003.12.013

Cheung, S., Tu, B., & Huang, C. (2022). Adverse childhood experiences, mindfulness, and grit in college students in China. *Frontiers in Psychology, 13*. https://doi.org/10.3389/fpsyg.2022.891532

Craig, S. L., Austin, A., Levenson, J. S., Leung, V. Y., Eaton, A. D., & D'Souza, S. F. (2020). Frequencies and patterns of adverse childhood events in LGBTQ+ youth. *Child Abuse & Neglect, 107*, 104623. https://doi.org/10.1016/j.chiabu.2020.104623

Credé, M., Tynan, M., & Harms, P. D. (2017). Much ado about grit: A meta-analytic synthesis of the grit literature. *Journal of Personality and Social Psychology, 113*(3), 492–511. https://doi.org/10.1037/pspp0000102

Datu, J. a. D. (2021). Beyond Passion and Perseverance: Review and future research initiatives on the science of grit. *Frontiers in Psychology, 11*. https://doi.org/10.3389/fpsyg.2020.545526

Dowling, B. A., Grigsby, T. J., Ziomek, G. J., & Schnarrs, P. W. (2023). Substance use outcomes for sexual and gender minority adults with a history of adverse childhood experiences: A scoping review. *Drug and Alcohol Dependence, 6*, 100129. https://doi.org/10.1016/j.dadr.2022.100129

Dube, S. R., Felitti, V. J., Dong, M., Chapman, D. P., Giles, W. H., & Anda, R. F. (2003). Childhood abuse, neglect, and household dysfunction and the risk of illicit drug use: The adverse childhood experiences study. *Pediatrics, 111*(3), 564–572. https://doi.org/10.1542/peds.111.3.564

Duckworth, A., Peterson, C., Matthews, M. D., & Kelly, D. R. (2007). Grit: Perseverance and passion for long-term goals. *Journal of Personality and Social Psychology, 92*(6), 1087–1101. https://doi.org/10.1037/0022-3514.92.6.1087

Duckworth, A. L., & Quinn, P. D. (2009). Development and validation of the short grit scale (Grit–S). *Journal of Personality Assessment, 91*(2), 166–174. https://doi.org/10.1080/00223890802634290

Eres, R., Postolovski, N., Thielking, M., & Lim, M. H. (2021). Loneliness, mental health, and social health indicators in LGBTQIA+ Australians. *American Journal of Orthopsychiatry, 91*(3), 358–366. https://doi.org/10.1037/ort0000531

Eskreis-Winkler, L., Shulman, E. P., Young, V. S., Tsukayama, E., Brunwasser, S. M., & Duckworth, A. L. (2016). Using wise interventions to motivate deliberate practice. *Journal of Personality and Social Psychology, 111*(5), 728–744. https://doi.org/10.1037/pspp0000074

Felitti, V. J., Anda, R. F., Nordenberg, D., Williamson, D. P., Spitz, A. M., Edwards, V. J., Koss, M. P., & Marks, J. G. (1998). Relationship of childhood abuse and household dysfunction to many of the leading causes of death in adults. *American Journal of Preventive Medicine, 14*(4), 245–258. https://doi.org/10.1016/s0749-3797(98)00017-8

Fish, J. N., Bishop, M. D., & Russell, S. T. (2023). Age trends in bias-based bullying and mental health by sexual orientation and gender identity. *Prevention Science, 24*(6), 1142–1151. https://doi.org/10.1007/s11121-023-01530-4

Friedman, M., Marshal, M. P., Guadamuz, T. E., Wei, C., Wong, C. F., Saewyc, E., & Stall, R. (2011). A meta-analysis of disparities in childhood sexual abuse, parental physical abuse, and peer victimization among sexual minority and sexual nonminority individuals. *American Journal of Public Health, 101*(8), 1481–1494. https://doi.org/10.2105/ajph.2009.190009

Frost, D. M., Lehavot, K., & Meyer, I. H. (2013). Minority stress and physical health among sexual minority individuals. *Journal of Behavioral Medicine*, *38*(1), 1–8. https://doi.org/10.1007/s10865-013-9523-8

Gardiner, B. (2018). Grit and stigma: Gay men ageing with HIV in regional Queensland. *Journal of Sociology*, *54*(2), 214–225. https://doi.org/10.1177/1440783318766162

Gomillion, S. C., & Giuliano, T. A. (2011). The influence of media role models on gay, lesbian, and bisexual identity. *Journal of Homosexuality*, *58*(3), 330–354. https://doi.org/10.1080/00918369.2011.546729

Hanif, R., Kliewer, W., & Riaz, R. (2022). Adverse childhood experiences, psychological well-being, and substance use in Pakistani university students. *South African Journal of Psychology*, 008124632211369. https://doi.org/10.1177/00812463221136958

Hatzenbuehler, M. L. (2010). Social factors as determinants of mental health disparities in LGB populations: Implications for public policy. *Social Issues and Policy Review*, *4*(1), 31–62. https://doi.org/10.1111/j.1751-2409.2010.01017.x

Herek, G. M., Gillis, J. R., & Cogan, J. C. (2009). Internalized stigma among sexual minority adults: Insights from a social psychological perspective. *Journal of Counseling Psychology*, *56*(1), 32–43. https://doi.org/10.1037/a0014672

Herrick, A. L., Stall, R., Chmiel, J. S., Guadamuz, T. E., Penniman, T. V., Shoptaw, S., Ostrow, D. G., & Plankey, M. (2013). It gets better: Resolution of internalized homophobia over time and associations with positive health outcomes among MSM. *AIDS and Behavior*, *17*(4), 1423–1430. https://doi.org/10.1007/s10461-012-0392-x

Huang, C., Tan, Y., Cheung, S., & Hu, H. (2021). Adverse childhood experiences and psychological well-being in Chinese college students: Mediation effect of mindfulness. *International Journal of Environmental Research and Public Health*, *18*(4), 1636. https://doi.org/10.3390/ijerph18041636

Institute of Medicine. (2011). *The health of lesbian, gay, bisexual, and transgender people: Building a foundation for better understanding*. National Academies Press.

Jin, J. S., & Kim, N. (2017). Grit, academic resilience, and psychological well-being in nursing students. *The Journal of Korean Academic Society of Nursing Education*, *23*(2), 175–183. https://doi.org/10.5977/jkasne.2017.23.2.175

Juda, E. (2021, April 15). *Confronting prejudice: How to protect yourself and help others | Pepperdine online California*. PEP-UMT. https://onlinegrad.pepperdine.edu/blog/prejudice-discrimination-coping-skills/

Khan, S. I., Hussain, M., Parveen, S., Bhuiyan, M. I., Gourab, G., Sarker, G., Arafat, S. M., & Sikder, J. (2009). Living on the extreme margin: Social exclusion of the transgender population (Hijra) in Bangladesh. *Journal of Health Population and Nutrition*, *27*(4). https://doi.org/10.3329/jhpn.v27i4.3388

Kosciw, J. G., et al. (2016). *The 2015 national school climate survey: The experiences of lesbian, gay, bisexual, transgender, and queer youth in our nation's schools*. GLSEN.

Lefevor, G. T., Huffman, C. E., & Blaber, I. P. (2020). Navigating potentially traumatic conservative religious environments as a Sexual/Gender minority. In *Springer eBooks* (pp. 317–329). https://doi.org/10.1007/978-3-030-52612-2_25

McCabe, S. E., Hughes, T. L., West, B. T., Evans-Polce, R. J., Veliz, P., Dickinson, K., & McCabe, V. V. (2020). Sexual orientation, adverse childhood experiences, and comorbid DSM-5 substance use and mental health disorders. *The Journal of Clinical Psychiatry*, *81*(6). https://doi.org/10.4088/jcp.20m13291

Meyer, I. H. (2003). Prejudice, social stress, and mental health in lesbian, gay, and bisexual populations: Conceptual issues and research evidence. *Psychological Bulletin*, *129*(5), 674–697. https://doi.org/10.1037/0033-2909.129.5.674

Pasha-Zaidi, N., Afari, E., Urganci, B., Sevi, B., & Durham, J. (2020). Investigating the relationship between adverse childhood experiences (ACEs) and resilience: A study of undergraduate students in Turkey. *Journal of Aggression, Maltreatment & Trauma, 29*(10), 1204–1221. https://doi.org/10.1080/10926771.2020.1725212

Richman, L. S., & Hatzenbuehler, M. L. (2014). A multilevel analysis of stigma and health. *Policy Insights from the Behavioral and Brain Sciences, 1*(1), 213–221. https://doi.org/10.1177/2372732214548862

Rogers, C. D. F., Pakdaman, S., Forster, M., Sussman, S., Grigsby, T. J., Victoria, J., & Unger, J. B. (2022). Effects of multiple adverse childhood experiences on substance use in young adults: A review of the literature. *Drug and Alcohol Dependence, 234*, 109407. https://doi.org/10.1016/j.drugalcdep.2022.109407

Röndahl, G., Innala, S., & Carlsson, M. (2006). Heterosexual assumptions in verbal and non-verbal communication in nursing. *Journal of Advanced Nursing, 56*(4), 373–381. https://doi.org/10.1111/j.1365-2648.2006.04018.x

Rosario, M., Rotheram-Borus, M. J., & Reid, H. M. (1996). Gay-related stress and its correlates among gay and bisexual male adolescents of predominantly Black and Hispanic background. *Journal of Community Psychology, 24*(2), 136–159. https://doi.org/10.1002/(sici)1520-6629(199604)24:2

Rusadi, R. M., Sugara, G. S., & Isti'adah, F. N. (2021). Effect of mindfulness-based cognitive therapy on academic grit among university student. *Current Psychology, 42*(6), 4620–4629. https://doi.org/10.1007/s12144-021-01795-4

Russell, G. M., & Richards, J. A. (2003). Stressor and resilience factors for lesbians, gay men, and bisexuals confronting antigay politics. *American Journal of Community Psychology, 31*(3–4), 313–328. https://doi.org/10.1023/a:1023919022811

Ryff, C. D. (1989). In search of Eudaimonia: The celebration of psychological well-being. *American Psychologist, 44*(6), 1617.

Ryff, C. D., & Keyes, C. L. M. (1995). The structure of psychological well-being revisited. *Journal of Personality and Social Psychology, 69*(4), 719–727. https://doi.org/10.1037/0022-3514.69.4.719

Schnarrs, P. W., Stone, A. L., Salcido, R., Baldwin, A., Georgiou, C., & Nemeroff, C. B. (2019). Differences in adverse childhood experiences (ACEs) and quality of physical and mental health between transgender and cisgender sexual minorities. *Journal of Psychiatric Research, 119*, 1–6. https://doi.org/10.1016/j.jpsychires.2019.09.001

Schilling, E. A., Aseltine, R. H., & Gore, S. (2007). Adverse childhood experiences and mental health in young adults: A longitudinal survey. *BMC Public Health, 7*(1). https://doi.org/10.1186/1471-2458-7-30

Schnarrs, P. W., Stone, A. L., Salcido, R., Georgiou, C., Zhou, X., & Nemeroff, C. B. (2020). The moderating effect of resilience on the relationship between adverse childhood experiences (ACEs) and quality of physical and mental health among adult sexual and gender minorities. *Behavioral Medicine, 46*(3–4), 366–374. https://doi.org/10.1080/08964289.2020.1727406

Shehzala, S., Jaiswal, A., Vemireddy, V., & Angeli, F. (2024). Social media "stars" vs "the ordinary" me: Influencer marketing and the role of self-discrepancies, perceived homophily, authenticity, self-acceptance and mindfulness. *European Journal of Marketing*. https://doi.org/10.1108/ejm-02-2023-0141

Shih, A. F., & Maroongroge, S. (2017). The importance of grit in medical training. *Journal of Graduate Medical Education, 9*(3), 399. https://doi.org/10.4300/jgme-d-16-00852.1

Sonu, S., Post, S. L., & Feinglass, J. (2019). Adverse childhood experiences and the onset of chronic disease in young adulthood. *Preventive Medicine, 123*, 163–170. https://doi.org/10.1016/j.ypmed.2019.03.032

Su, H., Wang, L., Li, Y., Yu, H., & Zhang, J. (2019). The mediating and moderating roles of self-acceptance and self-reported health in the relationship between self-worth and subjective well-being among elderly Chinese rural empty-nester. *Medicine*, *98*(28), e16149. https://doi.org/10.1097/md.0000000000016149

Thoits, P. A. (2011). Mechanisms linking social ties and support to physical and mental health. *Journal of Health and Social Behavior*, *52*(2), 145–161. https://doi.org/10.1177/0022146510395592

Vinothkumar, M., & Prasad, N. (2016). Moderating role of resilience in the relationship between grit and psychological well-being. *International Journal of Psychology and Psychiatry*, *4*(2), 10. https://doi.org/10.5958/2320-6233.2016.00009.2

12 Global Research Trends on Implementing Internet-Based Mental Health Programs

A Bibliometric Analysis

Mani Abdul Karim and Madalaimuthu Anthony

12.1 INTRODUCTION

Mental health conditions are often neglected in most countries across the globe. Because of this, the prevalence of mental health issues is drastically increasing today. According to a recent report by the World Health Organization (WHO), one person out of every eight is living with a condition of mental health disorder across the world.[1] Furthermore, 1 in every 200 adults suffers from Schizophrenia.[2] In addition, nearly a billion people worldwide live with a diagnosable mental disorder. To add to this severity, during and even post-COVID-19 pandemic period, there has been a high prevalence of certain psychiatric symptoms indicating disorders such as anxiety, post-traumatic stress, and depression; neurocognitive issues such as impaired attention, poor concentration, poor memory, and slow processing speed have also increased in patients with severe acute respiratory syndrome.[3] Due to this, the demand for counseling and psychological services has abruptly increased, particularly online or Internet-based mental health programs (I-MHP). Besides, a rise in disruptive technologies has made it possible to deliver mental health services using innovative approaches over digital mental health platforms. Ever-increasing AI-driven applications and ventures into the delivery of mental health care make it relevant to understand the patterns of mental health requirements, geographical demands, nature of mental health issues, and services required. The mapping of these thematic-based mental health programs would ensure an effective, individualized mental health program for the needy.

I-MHP have been found to be a most promising method to reduce various psychological symptoms and help to reach a wide range of people in a short span of time. Terminologically, it has been utilized interchangeably with a wide variety of phrases such as "e-mental health," "digital mental health,"[4] "Internet intervention,"[5] "tele

 DOI: 10.1201/9781003476344-12

mental health,"[6] and "online counseling." Internet-based interventions cover different types of psychological interventions which incorporate various psychotherapies and relaxation techniques: specifically, Internet-based cognitive behavior therapy (I-CBT and Internet-based mindfulness meditation (I-MM) are widely used in various psychological issues.[7,8] All these psychological interventions delivered across geographical boundaries through computer, smartphone, tablet, telephone, and other advanced modes of Internet-based communications.

Due to the wide range of utility of Internet-based interventions across various age groups, it is essential to identify the research hubs to understand the basic nature of trends for I-MHPs. Visual maps depicting the content and citations of published articles in the domain can provide insights to the readers with in-depth understanding of the research hubs and trends for potential future research direction. To our knowledge, there is no bibliometric review conducted in this domain, particularly in the context of I-MHPs till date. Bibliometric analysis can provide a visual presentation to synthesize the structural and evolutionary aspects of a research domain in its entirety, which is paramount for understanding and synthesizing the research advancements and directions in any field in a global context.[9-13]

12.2 METHODS

The data source was articles indexed by WoSCC database and the articles were extracted by using the searching algorithms to collate the dataset. TS in this context indicates Title Search.

Search Algorithm 1 (SET-1): ((((((((((TS=("e-mental health")) OR TS=(internet*)) OR TS= (Iot*)) OR TS=(IoMT*)) OR TS=("m-mental health)) OR TS=("digital mental health")) OR TS=("teleconferencing")) OR TS=("tele counselling") OR TS=("online counselling")) OR TS =("tele mental health")) OR TS=(tele-MH) OR TS=("video conferencing")) OR TS= ("internet intervention"). A total of 2,60,455 data were extracted using the above keywords. *Note:* IoT = Internet of Things; IoMT = Internet of Medical Things.

Search Algorithm 2 (SET-2): (((TS=("mental health")) OR TS=("psychological well-being")) OR TS=("psychosocial support"). A total of 3,04,618 data were extracted in this search strategy.

Search Algorithm 3: Combined SET 1 and 2 using "AND" Boolean.

Combined records of 7,134 data were taken for the bibliometric analysis by adding Strategy 1 and Strategy 2 between 1994 and 2023 (December 22, 2023). The PRISMA flowchart related to search strategy and sorting process of the extracted articles with criteria used for analysis in CiteSpace is shown in Figure 12.1.

12.3 RESULTS

As per the data depicted in Figure 12.2, there is a discernible upward trajectory in annual publications from 2020 and 2023, amounting to 3,766 publications, which represents more than half of the total publications. This signifies a consistent surge in research interest pertaining to Internet-based mental health programs during and

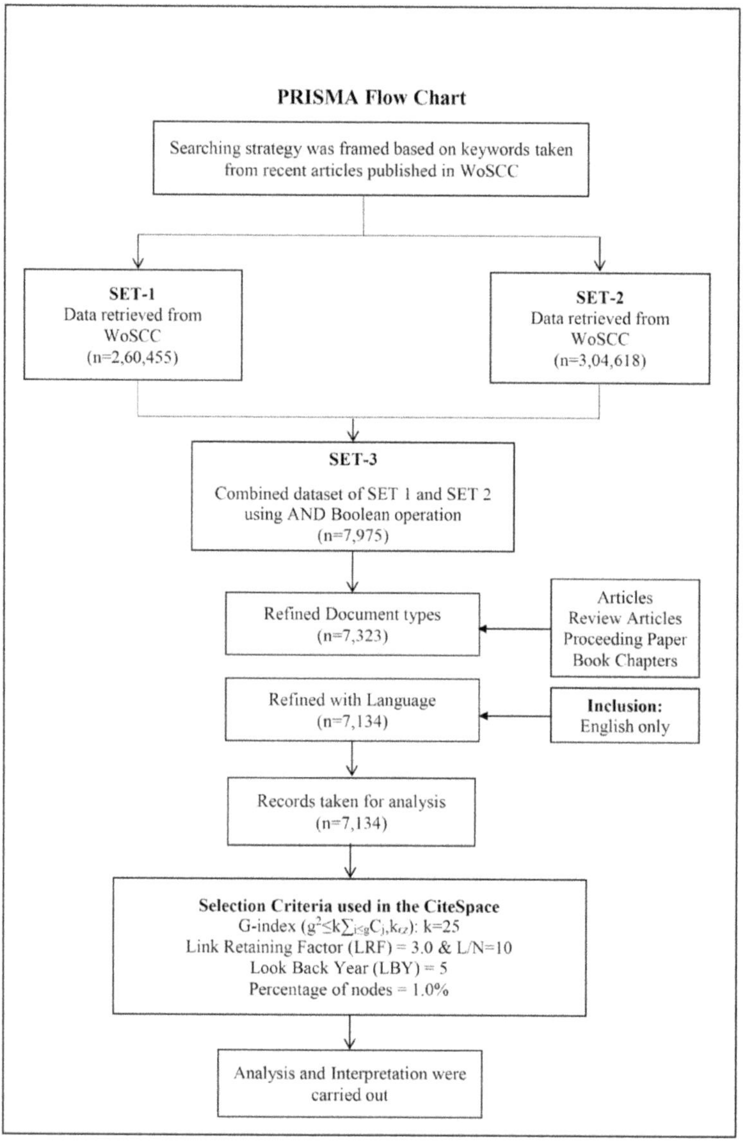

FIGURE 12.1 PRISMA flowchart for bibliometric analysis in CiteSpace on I-MHP.

post-COVID-19 pandemic. Preceding the year 2020, the advancement in implementing or researching alternative modalities for the delivery of counseling or psychological interventions was relatively limited.

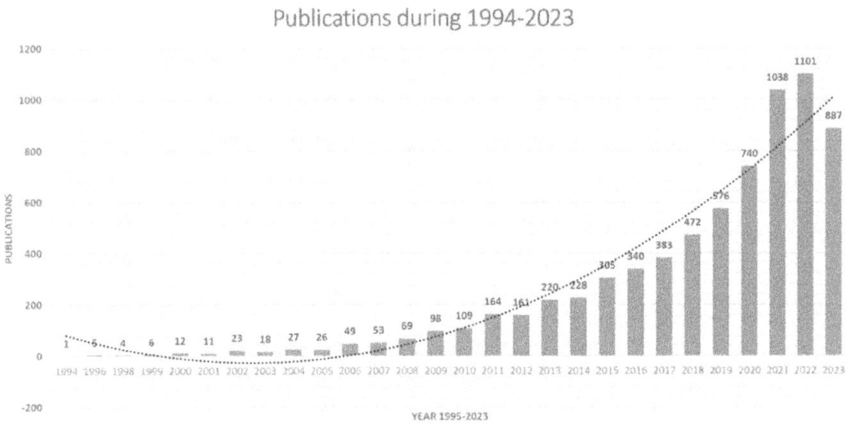

FIGURE 12.2 Annual publications on I-MHPs from 1994 to 2023.

12.3.1 Analysis of Countries/Regions

A total of 128 countries are involved in publications on several Internet-based mental health programs or interventions to mitigate various psychological issues. As shown in Table 12.1, the United States is on top in citation count (2,297), burst (109.43), and sigma (50.94). Based on centrality, India is on top (0.11) and it shows that the country influences more on bridging the network path between any two other nodes.

12.3.2 Analysis of Institutions

Figure 12.3 shows institutional network involved in most productive research on IMHP from 1994 to 2023. As shown in Table 12.2, the institution with the highest citation count was the University of London (287 publications), followed by the University of California System (233), Vrije Universiteit Amsterdam (217), Harvard University (215), and the University of Melbourne (191). The first institution in terms of centrality was Columbia University (0.09), followed by Harvard University (0.05), University of London (0.05), Johns Hopkins University (0.05), and Yale University (0.05). Based on Sigma ($\sum$) value, the first institution is Australian National University (2.10), followed by US Department of Veterans Affairs (1.43), Veterans Health Administration (VHA; 1.41), Columbia University (1.36), and Vrije Universiteit Amsterdam (1.34).

12.3.3 Predominant Publishers and Authors

Based on the list generated from Web of Science Core Collections, Elsevier was the top publisher which published 1,237 articles (17.34%), followed by Springer Nature (1,069; 14.98%), Jmir Publications (715; 10.02%), Wiley (529), and Frontiers Media (481; 6.74%).

TABLE 12.1
The Top Ten Countries on I-MHPs During 1994–2023

Rank	CC	Country	Burst	Country	σ	Country	Σ	Country
1	2,297	USA	109.43	USA	0.11	India	50.94	USA
2	1,028	Australia	17.40	The Netherlands	0.09	England	2.15	Australia
3	852	England	12.72	Australia	0.07	Scotland	1.89	The Netherlands
4	815	China	4.95	Denmark	0.06	Italy	1.16	Belgium
5	591	Germany	3.99	Pakistan	0.06	Saudi Arabia	1.15	Pakistan
6	559	Canada	3.91	Finland	0.06	South Africa	1.06	Finland
7	462	The Netherlands	3.90	Bangladesh	0.06	Australia	1.05	Denmark
8	252	Spain	3.49	Nigeria	0.06	UAE	1.05	Nigeria
9	234	Sweden	3.24	Belgium	0.05	Poland	1.01	Bangladesh
10	195	Japan	2.42	Gibraltar	0.05	Belgium	1.00	India

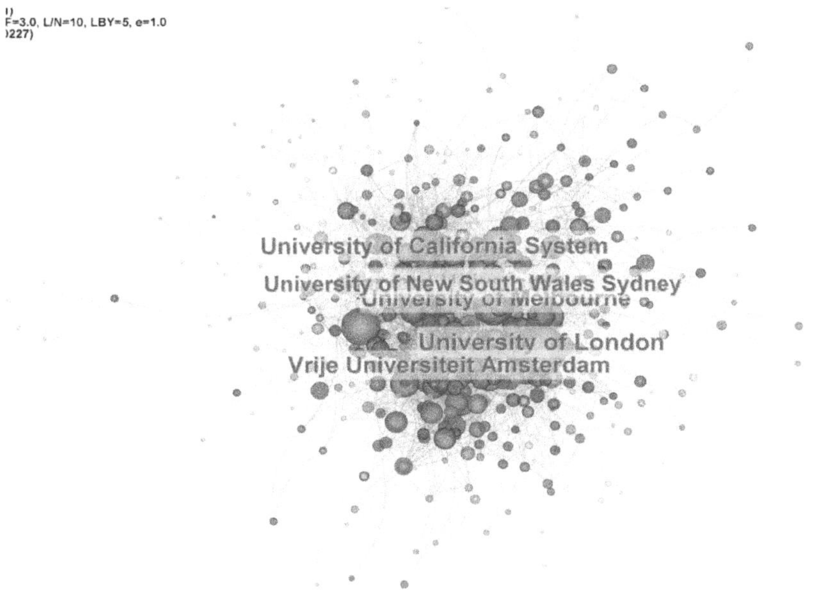

FIGURE 12.3 Institutional network analysis on I-MHPs from 1994 to 2023 using CiteSpace.

Among authors, Ebert, D.D. (101) had the highest number of publications, followed by Cuijpers, P. (88), Titov, N. (79), Baumeister, H. (72), Christensen, H. (71), Riper, H. (69), Andersson, G. (63), Dear, B.F. (60), Griffiths, M.D. (58), and Mohr, D.C. (47). Table 12.2 indicates top ten cited authors. Based on burst analysis, in the citation history of authors, Christensen, H. (2004) had the highest citation burst of 55.85, followed by Spek, V. (2008; 55.66), Griffiths, K.M. (2005; 43.98), Eysenbach, G. (2004; 39.71), Andersson, G. (2010; 33.34), and Barak, A. (2002; 31.43).

12.3.4 Co-Occurrences Keywords Analysis

This analysis is crucial for gaining insights into the evolving topics and trends within a specific field. It aids in understanding the progression of that particular area of study. Notably, the highest number of co-occurrences keywords based on frequency or citation count include "mental health" (2,915), followed by "depression" (1,477), "Internet" (1,190), "prevalence" (796), "anxiety" (782), and "adolescents" (656). Additionally, keywords with high centrality values include "mental health" (0.09), "Internet" (0.04), "life" (0.04), "adolescents" (0.03), and "primary care" (0.03). Identifying keywords with increased burst in citation indicates emerging trends in studies related to I-MHPs. Accordingly, the top five keywords with the highest burst values are "Internet" (29.76), "digital mental health" (20.90), "self-help" (18.24), "panic disorder" (17.58), and "digital health" (15.86).

TABLE 12.2
The Top Ten Cited Authors Published on I-MHPs between 1994 and 2023

Rank	CC	Author	Σ	Author	Σ	Author
1	4,354	Anonymous (1996)	0.12	Anonymous (1996)	2.00	Anonymous (1996)
2	906	Kessler, R.C. (2002)	0.08	Kraut, R. (2001)	1.69	Griffiths, M. (1999)
3	758	Kroenke, K. (2009)	0.07	Carlbring, P. (2004)	1.55	Kraut, R. (2001)
4	748	WHO (2005)	0.07	Griffiths, M. (1999)	1.53	Christensen, H. (2004)
5	726	Andersson G. (2006)	0.07	Beck, A.T. (1999)	1.48	Spek, V. (2008)
6	608	Cuijpers, P. (2008)	0.05	Andrews, G. (2004)	1.33	Klein, B. (2002)
7	607	Christensen, H. (2004)	0.05	Cuijpers, P. (2008)	1.29	Eysenbach, G. (2004)
8	580	Soitzer, R.L. (2009)	0.05	Young, K.S. (2002)	1.24	Barak, A. (2002)
9	499	Eysenbach, G. (2004)	0.05	APA (2004)	1.23	Carlbring, P. (2004)
10	489	Andrews, G. (2004)	0.04	Andersson, G. (2006)	1.22	Clarke, G. (2006)

12.3.5 Inter-Document Citation Network Analysis

The analysis revealed a total of 20 separate clusters within the co-cited document analysis network. The visualization map of DCA-based clusters is shown in Figure 12.4 and the top five most cited articles related to I-MHPs are presented in Table 12.3. Table 12.3 provides an overview of the significance and citation count of the top 5 clusters out of the total 20. These clusters represent distinct interventions that were implemented and actively researched in Internet-based mental health programs from 1994 to 2023. Figure 12.4 visually emphasizes several key clusters within the DCA network. Particularly, the network demonstrated a substantial weighted mean silhouette value of 0.9075, indicating a significant level of homogeneity within the clusters.

Table 12.3 also exhibits more specific insights, revealing silhouette values within the range of 0.819–0.938 for the top five clusters in DCA analysis. These values distinctly indicate a notable degree of uniformity observed within each cluster. Additionally, the mean year of the top five clusters spans from 2010 to 2019. able 12.3 also contains a succinct compilation of crucial data elements.

12.4 DISCUSSION

The examination of annual publications revealed general upswing post-2010. Specifically, within the recent four years (2019–2023), there were 3,766 records published, surpassing half the total publications from the preceding 25 years (1994–2019). This surge indicates a significant increase in the utilization of the Internet

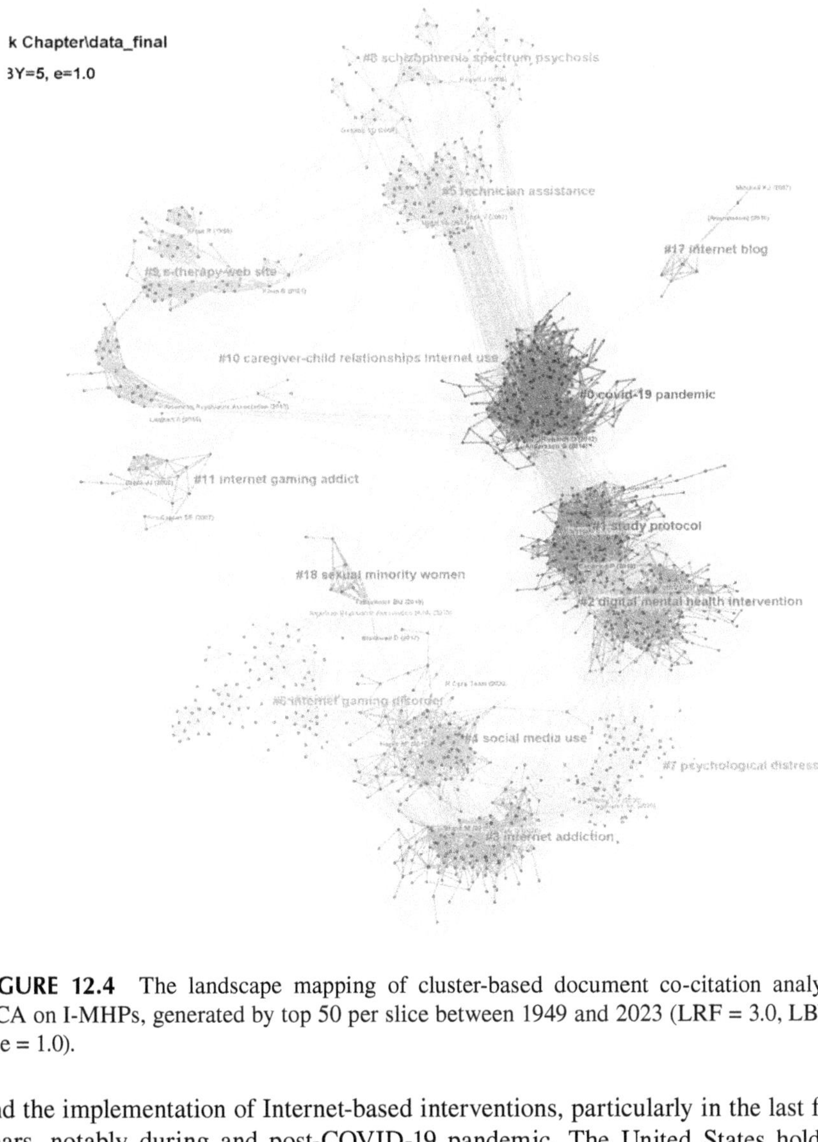

FIGURE 12.4 The landscape mapping of cluster-based document co-citation analysis: DCA on I-MHPs, generated by top 50 per slice between 1949 and 2023 (LRF = 3.0, LBY = 5, e = 1.0).

and the implementation of Internet-based interventions, particularly in the last four years, notably during and post-COVID-19 pandemic. The United States holds a predominant position in terms of citation counts (2,297), burst (109.43), and sigma (50.94). However, India leads in terms of betweenness centrality (0.11).

Among the top five most productive institutions, the University of London secures a top position in both citation count (287) and centrality (0.05), while Colombia University features in the top five for both centrality (0.09) and sigma (1.36). An analysis of keyword co-occurrences, focusing on recent burst, reveals that keywords such as "Internet," "digital mental health," "self-help," "panic disorder," and "digital health" serve as indicators for emerging trends in this domain.

TABLE 12.3
The Five DCA Clusters with First Five Oft-Cited References Ranked by Counts of Citation

Cluster #	Cluster Size	Silhouette Value	Mean (Year)	Cc	Burst	Σ	∑	DOI of Cited References
0	255	0.819	2010	90	33.90	0.01	1.41	10.1002/wps.20083
COVID-19				86	43.34	0.07	16.63	10.1016/j.cpr.2012.02.004
pandemic				63	35.40	0.04	3.92	10.1371/journal.pone.0013196
				62	35.76	0.03	2.78	10.1080/16506070903318960
				44	24.44	0.00	1.00	10.2196/jmir.1923
1	195	0.913	2015	190	7.76	0.03	1.29	10.1080/16506073.2017.1401115
Study protocol				133	15.21	0.04	1.72	10.1001/jamapsychiatry.2017.0044
				105	4.93	0.03	1.15	10.1027/1016-9040/a000318
				93	38.26	0.03	3.30	10.1002/wps.20151
				83	7.76	0.01	1.08	10.1016/j.jad.2017.07.021
2	194	0.868	2017	145	15.49	0.02	1.32	10.1016/j.janxdis.2018.01.001
Digital mental				88	12.34	0.02	1.26	10.1002/wps.20472
health				74	7.25	0.00	1.02	10.1002/wps.20610
				74	0.00	0.00	1.00	10.1001/jamapsychiatry.2020.4364
				67	10.96	0.01	1.14	10.1016/j.jad.2017.04.046
3	134	0.905	2019	64	17.29	0.01	1.24	10.1016/j.comppsych.2020.152180
Internet				52	14.03	0.00	1.04	10.1016/j.neubiorev.2019.06.032
addiction				48	12.95	0.00	1.04	10.1556/2006.2020.00016
				44	11.86	0.00	1.03	10.3389/fpsyt.2020.00751
				41	11.05	0.00	1.01	10.1001/jamanetworkopen.2020.19686
4	123	0.938	2016	129	0.00	0.00	1.00	–
Social media				68	9.84	0.01	1.10	–
use				64	12.59	0.03	1.47	10.1037/adb0000160
				57	9.55	0.01	1.12	10.1016/j.jad.2016.08.030
				53	8.17	0.01	1.08	10.1080/02673843.2019.1590851

Outstanding research articles that have significantly contributed to innovation and advancements in e-mental health are identified based on the number of citations. DCA analysis has revealed 20 clusters, each associated with distinct implications for Internet-based mental health programs across various psychological issues. Within these clusters, two can be identified as emerging trends and hubs in this research area based on the mean year of the cluster—Cluster #2 (digital mental health) and Cluster #3 (Internet addiction).

Cluster #0 (COVID-19 pandemic) predominantly focuses on the implementation of I-MHPs for conditions like depression, anxiety, and various psychiatric disorders. Study findings highlight the potential efficacy of Internet-delivered treatments and computerized treatments for depression, suggesting their viability as evidence-based approaches.[14,15] Several research works have emphasized the effectiveness of Internet-based cognitive behavior therapy (iCBT) as a promising treatment, widely employed through computers and the Internet to address psychiatric disorders and other clinical problems.[7,16–18] Numerous advantages have been identified in the use of I-MHPs, including cost-effectiveness, enhanced accessibility, the ability to tailor content based on symptoms or severity, the transition from easy to challenging training difficulties, and the capacity for self-improvement in the comfort of one's home. Additionally, interventions delivered through the web-based or mobile platform, often termed eHealth/mHealth interventions, represent alternative tools or treatment methods adapted and operationalized for delivery through the Internet or mobile platforms.[19, 20]

Cluster #1 yields mean year of 2015 with cluster size of 195. This is intensive on iCBT, a robust way to address some of the shortcomings in traditional therapy. There are various clinical trials that have demonstrated the effectiveness of iCBT in treating anxiety, stress, depression, and insomnia.[17,21] This iCBT treatment protocol incorporates several advantages, including individuals to access this Internet intervention from any place regardless of their geographical location, engage in iCBT at a time that suits their schedule, and develop coping skills and strategies.[16,18,22]

Another cluster (Cluster #2; digital mental health) predominantly occupied with digital mental health and the cluster size is 194, with silhouette value of 0.868, and the mean year for it is 2017. Digital mental health interventions utilize various digital technologies, such as mobile apps, online counseling, tele-therapy, tablet, wearables and sensors, chatbots and virtual assistants, and online support communities, to deliver mental health services or support.[4, 21, 23–26] This emerging field leverages technology to increase access to mental health resources, provide timely assistance, and facilitate the delivery of evidence-based interventions.

Cluster #3 (Internet addiction) is specifically about the themes related to Internet addiction (size of cluster is 134, with silhouette value 0.905 and mean year 2019). In this cluster, most of the articles studied about Internet addiction, specifically gaming disorder and problematic Internet usage (PIU). PIU is a condition where individuals experience excessive, compulsive, or harmful patterns of Internet use that interfere with their everyday life routines, interpersonal relationships, and overall psychological well-being. After COVID-19 pandemic, the use of digital application increased drastically in all the domains of life. Various studies pointed out the negative impact of Internet gaming or problematic Internet use among various age groups, including children, adolescents, and youth.[27–30] Though various Internet-based interventions help individuals to come out of various psychological issues, there are some common negative effects associated with Internet use, including addiction and compulsive behavior, social isolation, sleep disturbances, impact on academic and occupational functioning, impact on relationships, physical health illness, and information overload.

12.4.1 Implications for Future Research in I-MHPs

The bibliometric results provide several implications for future research directions in I-MHPs. The use of Internet-based mental health programs, by and large, has increased rigorously after the COVID-19 pandemic. Notably, the implementation of iCBT in various psychosocial issues among children, adolescents, and older adults is clearly visible. However, future research on integrating module like combination of iCBT and mindfulness or iCBT and psychotherapy is much warranted to enhance its outcomes. Furthermore, there are less number of studies done in Internet-based mindfulness and Internet-based psychotherapy as compared to iCBT. Therefore, conducting such research is needed to enhance the empirical evidence of those therapies for all age groups.

12.5 CONCLUSIONS

This bibliometric study aimed to gain insights into the global landscape of Internet-based mental health programs during 1994–2023. A noteworthy observation is that over half of the total publications emerged during and after the COVID-19 pandemic, indicating a substantial surge in research interest surrounding the implementation of I-MHPs. The United States has played a very significant role in the field of I-MHP, securing the top position based on citation count (2,297), burst (109.43), and sigma value (50.94). Despite India leading in terms of betweenness centrality (0.11), research activity in this domain is relatively limited. Digital mental health and Internet addiction emerged as prominent clusters in the field, as revealed by the DCA analysis. This study contributes valuable insights into Internet-based psychological interventions, shedding light on research achievements, collaborative networks among countries and institutions, and frequently cited documents. Future research directions should prioritize addressing the negative effects of Internet use across all age groups, with a specific focus on mitigating these effects among individuals.

REFERENCES

1. WHO. *World Mental Health Report: Transforming Mental Health for All.* WHO; 2022. DOI: 10.1136/bmj.o1593.
2. Tsuang MT, Faraone SV, Glatt SJ. *Schizophrenia.* 3rd ed. Oxford University Press: Oxford University Press; 2011.

3. Kathirvel N. Post COVID-19 pandemic mental health challenges. *Asian J Psychiatr* 2020; 53. DOI: 10.1016/j.ajp.2020.102430.
4. Hollis C, Falconer CJ, Martin JL, et al. Annual research review: digital health interventions for children and young people with mental health problems – a systematic and meta-review. *J Child Psychol Psychiatry Allied Discip* 2017; 58: 474–503.
5. Andersson G, Titov N, Dear BF, et al. Internet-delivered psychological treatments: from innovation to implementation. *World Psychiatry* 2019; 18: 20–28.
6. Abraham A, Jithesh A, Doraiswamy S, et al. Telemental health use in the COVID-19 pandemic: a scoping review and evidence gap mapping. *Front Psychiatry* 2021; 12: 1–16.
7. Karyotaki E, Efthimiou O, Miguel C, et al. Internet-based cognitive behavioral therapy for depression: a systematic review and individual patient data network meta-analysis. *JAMA Psychiatry* 2021; 78: 361–371.
8. Dworschak C, Heim E, Maercker A. Efficacy of internet-based interventions for common mental disorder symptoms and psychosocial problems in older adults: a systematic review and meta-analysis. *Internet Interv* 2022; 27: 100498.
9. Chen C, Chen Y, Horowitz M, et al. Towards an explanatory and computational theory of scientific discovery. *J Informetr* 2009; 3: 191–209.
10. Chen C. Searching for intellectual turning points: progressive knowledge domain visualization. *Proc Natl Acad Sci U S A* 2004; 101: 5303–5310.
11. Karim MA, Venkatachalam J. Global trends on studies with cognitive training: Mapping and bibliometric analysis using CiteSpace. *Cogn Brain, Behav An Interdiscip J* 2021; 25: 311–340.
12. Chen C, Ibekwe-SanJuan F, Hou J. The structure and dynamics of cocitation clusters: a multiple-perspective cocitation analysis. *J Am Soc Inf Sci Technol* 2010; 61: 1386–1409.
13. Rousseeuw PJ. Silhouettes: a graphical aid to the interpretation and validation of cluster analysis. *J Comput Appl Math* 1987; 20: 53–65.
14. Andersson G, Cuijpers P. Internet-based and other computerized psychological treatments for adult depression: a meta-analysis. *Cogn Behav Ther* 2009; 38: 196–205.
15. Andersson G, Titov N. Advantages and limitations of Internet-based interventions for common mental disorders. *World Psychiatry* 2014; 13: 4–11.
16. Titov N, Andrews G, Davies M, et al. Internet treatment for depression: a randomized controlled trial comparing clinician vs. technician assistance. *PLoS One* 2010; 5: 1–9.
17. Carlbring P, Andersson G, Cuijpers P, et al. Internet-based vs. face-to-face cognitive behavior therapy for psychiatric and somatic disorders: an updated systematic review and meta-analysis. *Cogn Behav Ther* 2018; 47: 1–18.
18. Titov N, Dear B, Nielssen O, et al. ICBT in routine care: a descriptive analysis of successful clinics in five countries. *Internet Interv* 2018; 13: 108–115.
19. Eysenbach G, Stoner S, Drozd F, et al. ConSORT-eHealth: improving and standardizing evaluation reports of web-based and mobile health interventions. *J Med Internet Res* 2011; 13. DOI: 10.2196/jmir.1923.
20. Boogerd E, Maas-Van Schaaijk NM, Sas TC, et al. Sugarsquare, a Web-based patient portal for parents of a child with type 1 diabetes: multicenter randomized controlled feasibility trial. *J Med Internet Res* 2017; 19: 1–8.
21. Andrews G, Basu A, Cuijpers P, et al. Computer therapy for the anxiety and depression disorders is effective, acceptable and practical health care: an updated meta-analysis. *J Anxiety Disord* 2018; 55: 70–78.
22. Carlbring P, Andersson G, Cuijpers P, et al. Internet-based vs. face-to-face cognitive behavior therapy for psychiatric and somatic disorders: an updated systematic review and meta-analysis. *Cogn Behav Ther* 2018; 47: 1–18.

23. Torous J, Firth J. Bridging the dichotomy of actual versus aspirational digital health. *World Psychiatry* 2018; 17: 108–109.
24. Torous J, Nicholas J, Larsen ME, et al. Clinical review of user engagement with mental health smartphone apps: evidence, theory and improvements. *Evid Based Ment Health* 2018; 21: 116–119.
25. Linardon J, Cuijpers P, Carlbring P, et al. The efficacy of app-supported smartphone interventions for mental health problems: a meta-analysis of randomized controlled trials. *World Psychiatry* 2019; 18: 325–336.
26. Firth J, Torous J, Nicholas J, et al. Can smartphone mental health interventions reduce symptoms of anxiety? A meta-analysis of randomized controlled trials. *J Affect Disord* 2017; 218: 15–22.
27. Dong H, Yang F, Lu X, et al. Internet addiction and related psychological factors among children and adolescents in China during the coronavirus disease 2019 (COVID-19) epidemic. *Front Psychiatry* 2020; 11: 1–9.
28. Sohn SY, Rees P, Wildridge B, et al. Correction to: prevalence of problematic smartphone usage and associated mental health outcomes amongst children and young people: a systematic review, meta-analysis and GRADE of the evidence (BMC Psychiatry 2019; 19(1): 356. DOI: 10.1186/s12888-019-2350). *BMC Psychiatry* 2021; 21: 1–10.
29. King DL, Delfabbro PH, Billieux J, et al. Problematic online gaming and the COVID-19 pandemic. *J Behav Addict* 2020; 9: 184–186.
30. Oka T, Hamamura T, Miyake Y, et al. Prevalence and risk factors of internet gaming disorder and problematic internet use before and during the COVID-19 pandemic: a large online survey of Japanese adults. *J Psychiatr Res* 2021; 142: 218–225.

13 Transformative Tales

Unveiling Success Stories and Advancements in Healthcare through Internet of Medical Things (IoMT) and Machine Learning Integration

Suresh Babu C.V. and Suruthi G.

13.1 INTRODUCTION

13.1.1 Contribution of IoMT in Healthcare

IoMT has contributed too many success stories and advancements in healthcare. Healthcare plays a significant role in safeguarding individual and public health. This led to the immediate urge for developing a technology for remote monitoring, automating data collection, analysis, and communication which in turn could contribute to cost reduction and patient empowerment. In order to achieve this, healthcare provider and companies started exploring ways to leverage connected devices for monitoring, diagnosis, and treatment. In early stages (1970–1980), remote monitoring systems and medical telemetry were developed to enhance healthcare domain. Later, during the 1990s and early 2000s, Internet of Things (IoT) marked its place in developing technology and grabbed attention of many and it also turned out to be the basement of IoMT. The advancements in sensor technology enabled the interconnectivity of data and devices and it was coined as IoT (Merchant, 2024). In case of IoMT, it all started in the early 2010s when the healthcare providers and many companies began exploring the application of IoT principles to healthcare, giving rise to IoMT. Some of the applications of IoMT involve regulatory landscape (FDA in the United States), data analytics with AI, and so on (Lutkevich & DelVecchio, 2024).

DOI: 10.1201/9781003476344-13

13.1.2 Interdependency of IoMT and ML as a Basement for Success Stories

Some experts have quoted on IoMT as "Internet of Medical Things holds immense potential to revolutionize healthcare by facilitating remote monitoring, personalized treatments, and improved patient outcomes. However, ensuring data security, interoperability, and regulatory compliance are critical challenges that must be addressed to fully realize its benefits." Machine learning, a subdomain of AI, took shape during the 1950s–1960s. ML has been known for the development of algorithms and statistical models that enables computers to perform task without the need for explicit programming. ML majorly contributed self- learning data and prediction or decision-based learning (Firican, 2024). These trends of ML were the reason for their adaptation in IoMT. IoMT is highly dependent on ML for analyzing the generated health-related data through connected devices by the use of ML algorithms. In other words, ML algorithms are used to analyze the data generated by a device or network to extract meaningful insights and improve healthcare outcomes (Suresh Babu & Praveen, 2023). The outcome of integration of IoMT and ML results in a data-driven and more personalized approach to healthcare, fostering finer patient outcomes and more efficient healthcare delivery.

13.1.3 Scope of the Study

This study aims to unleash the backstories and base reasons for the success and advancement of IoMT in healthcare, focusing on case studies, key features of IoMT, and advantages of IoMT over other technologies under the domain of healthcare. In addition, highlighted news on success and failure of IoMT will be provided with the key reasons for either their failure or success (Suresh Babu, C. V., Akkash Anniyappa et al., 2024). Along with this, we target to provide in-depth vision on improvising the IoMT technology by bridging the gap between the success and advancement through real-world incidents that grabbed attention of many companies, researchers, and market.

13.1.4 Objectives of the Study

The primary aims of this study are as follows:

1. Unveil the success stories and advancements in healthcare through IoMT with real incidents and case studies as the center of attraction.
2. Identify the wealth of IoMT over other existing technologies.
3. Unleash the key reasons and backstories of IoMT's success stories and advancements.
4. Proposing future research direction and recommendations for maximizing the benefits of IoMT in integration with ML.

13.2 LITERATURE REVIEW

13.2.1 Overview of IoMT

The healthcare sector relies heavily on the Internet of Things, which allows connected medical devices to monitor biological signals in order to diagnose illnesses without the need for human intervention (Vishnu et al., 2020). IoMT combines IoT and medical devices making strong implications in improving the quality of healthcare systems. IoMT allied mobile health services, remote healthcare, smart hospitals, and enhanced chronic illness management woes the implication of IoMT in the improvement of the quality of healthcare (Razdan et al., 2022). Many claim that the one great limitation of health personnel is the number of patients seen efficiently, but with IoMT's capability to improve efficiency by automating repetitive operations, physicians will be able to attend to more patients (Vishnu et al., 2020).

13.2.2 Impact of IoMT in HealthCare

The Internet of Medical Things is a focus of entrepreneurs in the health sector as it is an asset for enhancing service delivery by being quick and efficient while elevating the patient's health. However, its business plans for profitability as a potential of creating jobs has its own risk in data security. Organizations should not take this lightly as it endangers employees' lives and the privacy of the data (Giri et al., 2019). For example, during the COVID-19 pandemic, IoMT devices, applications, and communication protocols were widely criticized because their main purpose was to trace and help identify infected people. But there are more serious threats posed by these systems, such as their effect on everyday life. Other applications of IoMT such as device detection, monitoring, and testing are more alarming (Shakeel et al., 2023).

13.2.3 Benefits of IoMT

The healthcare sector is being revolutionized by the Internet of Medical Things, which links medical systems and devices to the Internet. It provides advantages like enhanced productivity and better patient care. Early detection of health problems is made possible by the real-time monitoring of vital signs. Telemedicine improves access to care and decreases in-person visits, particularly in impoverished areas. Healthcare personnel can concentrate on providing high-quality care since IoMT devices automate inventory management and patient data collection. Personalized care and better results are made possible by the insightful insights that IoMT data analytics offer into population health patterns (Thaploo, 2023).

13.2.4 Challenges Faced in IoMT

Despite its youth, IoMT technology presents security risks because of low user awareness, poor maintenance, and inadequate standards (Suresh Babu et al., 2024). IoMT devices with weak security are easily taken over by hackers, and they can use ransomware to access unencrypted IoMT devices via unencrypted communication (Kamalov et al., 2023). The critical security threats of IoMT greatly impact the confidentiality, integrity, authenticity, and availability of its data and associated resources (Garg et al., 2022).

13.2.5 Applications of IoMT in Healthcare

IoMT has set its benchmark in healthcare by improvising workflows, preventive care, and patient outcomes. It includes telemedicine platforms, smart implants, wearable technology, and management systems (Shakeel et al., 2023). IoMT technology makes wearable sensors, portable devices, and medical equipment more utilitarian, affordable, and proficient in tracking patients health, collecting clinical data, prognosticating diseases, and notifying users to emergencies (Dwivedi et al., 2022).

13.2.6 Privacy and Security Factor in IoMT

Unencrypted traffic constitutes critical security risks in the IoMT sector, which contributes to 57% of devices being vulnerable to sensitive data attacks. Strict privacy regulations must be implemented and cryptographic or non-cryptographic algorithms are highly recommended for implementation to ensure intrusion detection and prevention (Shakeel et al., 2023). Blockchain technology and AI are crucial for a secure financial industry, with IoMT systems facilitating information sharing and AI identifying anomalies in network traffic and patient data (Hireche et al., 2022).

13.2.7 Advancement of IoMT in Healthcare

A novel strategy for IoMT advancement is the incorporation of ML, AI, 5G, and IoT technologies in healthcare research. However, because of the difficulties with data security, privacy, transfer learning, and interoperability, successful integration is happening slowly. Encryption techniques like AES, ABE, and PDP can be used to protect data, but their efficacy depends on the specific conditions in which they are applied (Shafiq et al., 2024).

13.2.7.1 IoMT Setting Benchmarks (Highlighted News)

"Internet of medical things (IoMT) in e-clinics: enabling connected healthcare in smart cities."

Integrating public safety, emergency services, social services, housing quality, environmental health, and transportation can revolutionize the healthcare industry in a smart city. Medical professionals can receive better care, recuperate more quickly, and save money, thanks to the Internet of Medical Things (IoMT). Early intervention is made possible by connected systems that watch, alert, and alarm carers and providers (Thaploo, 2023).

"Safeguarding IoMT and connected devices is an ongoing challenge."

Henry Ford Health's director of medical device and IoT security expressed optimism despite challenges like in-depth scans and legacy software risks, citing increased manufacturer accountability and new FDA regulations (Miliard, 2023).

"Transforming Healthcare through IoMT Firmware Development."

The Internet of Things and its specialized offshoot, the Internet of Medical Things, have significantly advanced healthcare. For successful IoT development, there is an urging necessity for the integration of other technical factors, including embedded solutions and firmware development. These factors ensure secure data transmission between devices and healthcare systems which in turn enable seamless integration of medical devices, sensors, and wearables within the IoT network. This improves diagnosis and treatment through remote patient monitoring (IoT, Business News, 2023).

13.2.8 Future Trends of IoMT

The future of IoMT in healthcare impacts the growth of advancing technologies. The advancement and increasing demand for personalized healthcare and remote monitoring positions the growth of IoMT in healthcare. Additionally, the improvising of security and privacy issues would contribute to the success stories of IoMT in healthcare (Kamalov et al., 2023). The criticality of medical data greatly imposes the need for accuracy and security (Srivastava et al., 2022). Quantum systems, 5G, and quantum systems will be the main topics of future IoMT research. Investigations into security flaws, causes, and solutions related to remote cryptography key exploitation will be carried out (Sadhu et al., 2022).

13.3 THEORETICAL FRAMEWORK

13.3.1 Machine Learning and IoMT Integration

This study provides insights into the integration of IoT and ML resulting in the hybrid approach toward IoMT. IoT devices generate a richest outcome of real-time data wherein the ML algorithms process and analyze this data to provide enriched result leading to success stories. IoMT collaboration with ML has greater impact on healthcare industry by improving the performance and maximizing the efficiency (Nigar et al., 2023).

13.3.2 Selection of IoMT and Machine Learning over Other Technologies

ML plays a dominant role in the smart and automated strategies to make life easier. ML has been able to influence its benefit over healthcare industry through smart technologies, from smallest applications like wearable devices, smart thermometers, and RPM machines to bigger applications like robotic surgery. The ML algorithms increase the performance and adaptability of IoT devices in real-world scenario, making IoMT and ML preferable and effective over other technologies (Ordr, 2024).

13.3.3 Conceptual Definition

In this study, IoMT is defined as the network of medical devices, software, and services that are connected to healthcare information along the adaptability feature to evolving real-time data through ML algorithms. ML refers to algorithms that influence health information resulting in a precise output.

13.3.4 Theoretical Constructs and Relationships

The integrated framework of IoMT and ML outcasted its performance in the domain of healthcare with its promising results and success stories. The most basic and affordable IoMT device is wearable device like smartwatches that collect healthcare data such as body temperature and blood pressure without human intervention ("bgosoftware", 2024).

13.3.5 Integration with Literature Review

This theoretical framework on evolution of IoMT and incorporation of ML in IoMT has been influenced by previous researches done by various researchers and this is follow-up to unveil the success stories that surpassed the evolution of IoMT from its initial to this phase which almost occupied all headlines and flooded into domain of healthcare with its exclusive results (Thaploo, 2023).

13.3.6 Limitations and Assumption

The theoretical framework on collaboration of IoMT and ML leading to success stories has its own limitations when the topic of security involves. The security has been the greatest threat in journey of IoMT evolution (Kamalov et al., 2023). There were many data breaches and attacks like ransomware that had great impact on basic triads of security: confidentiality, integrity, and authenticity and availability (Garg et al., 2022).

13.3.7 Alignment with Research Design

The theoretical framework informs the selection of research methods, including surveys, newsletters, and observational studies, to explore the factors influencing IoMT adoption in integration with ML among healthcare providers and patients. Furthermore, the theoretical frameworks unleash the research findings and development of recommendations for fostering IoMT integration in healthcare along with techniques that could mitigate this security issue. In addition, success stories of IoMT have been the main lead of the plot.

13.3.8 Concluding Remarks

As concluding remarks, the IoMT has captured its place in healthcare industry along with ML with its divine contribution to success stories by improving efficiency in healthcare, lessening the burden on medical specialist, enhancing the result with technology-based diagnosis, and mitigating the issues caused by human errors. This study focuses on the success stories of IoMT in healthcare along with reasons behind this success events. In addition, an overview of security side of IoMT and discussion on research findings on improvising security have been provided.

13.4 RESEARCH METHODOLOGY

13.4.1 Introduction to Research Methodology

The current ruling technologies of IoMT and ML have great influence on healthcare in improving quality and accuracy by connecting patients, doctors, and medical devices, including hospital equipment, diagnostic gear, and wearable technology by transmitting information over a secure network (Watts, 2023). This study unleashes the key reasons behind the advancement in the healthcare domain. In addition, a comparative analysis of traditional approach (manual) and modern approach (technology-based) has been provided.

13.4.2 Research Design

This study focuses on the potency outcome achieved through integration of IoMT and ML, where various methodologies play important roles in advancing healthcare and its applications. One well-known methodology is sensor data fusion which involves blending data from numerous IoMT devices such as wearable sensors, medical implants, and mobile health apps. This merging data enables diversified patient monitoring and provides an encompassing view of individual health status. Preprocessing and extraction of relevant features from raw sensor data is done using technique called signal processing which facilitates ML analysis (Brena et al., 2020). A widely used learning, federated learning, is promising for securely protecting data during training machine learning models across IoMT devices, which increases the confidentiality and availability of data (Prasad et al., 2023). Nonetheless, explainable ML strategies are aimed at enhancing the comprehensibility of machine learning models. Physicians ought to believe in the effectiveness of IoMT- and ML-derived recommendations.

13.4.3 Sampling Strategy

These methods have contributed to IoMT and ML integrated devices which aid in the early diagnosis of diseases, enhance the patients' health, and provide healthcare that is tailored to the individual. Combining IoMT devices with machine learning models in an organized manner ensures that the devices perform in the best possible way regarding healthcare applications. The procedure begins with the first stage of the process whereby specialized IoMT devices are able to capture real-time data on patients, which is also run through ML algorithms for analyzing and preprocessing. The algorithms then go on to define the outliers within the data, position the patients' inputs, and alter their respective treatment plans. All of these models are evaluated in the same way with parameters like characteristics state, feasibility measure, and health representation parameters enhancing the credibility of all. After validation, the models are redistributed to IoMT devices where improved patient outcomes, practical recommendations, and support with clinical decision-making are performed. This methodology depends on clinical IoMT and ML systems that are never fully complete and always in a developmental stage to broaden the scope of healthcare technology.

13.4.4 Data Collection Methods

There are various steps involved in combining IoMT devices with ML techniques to gather data. The collection of medical data is made through wearables, sensors, or medical imaging tools. IoMT devices consist of data such as vital signs, patient activity, and environmental parameters. The complex data structures are handled by advanced ML techniques like deep learning, which increase predictive modeling tasks' correctness. On the other hand, patient privacy which is considered as vital and adherence to legal requirements such as HIPAA are guaranteed by data anonymization and encryption. Most commonly used technique is sensor data collection, where IoMT devices furnished with sensors such as accelerometers, gyroscopes, or temperature sensors capture physiological and environmental real-time data. This data lay out valuable insights into patient health status or environmental conditions. Additionally, electronic health records (EHRs) incorporation facilitates the collection of historical patient data which in return enables ML algorithms to learn from past trends and patterns. If we look into wearable devices, such as smartwatches or fitness trackers, we find they greatly contribute to data collection by continuously monitoring vital signs or activity levels. In addition, imaging techniques like MRI and CT scans generate rich medical data for ML algorithms which could be used for analyzing of diagnosis and assist in treatment. Overall, the synergy between IoMT and ML relies on diverse data collection techniques to yield eclectic insights for improved healthcare outcomes (Giri et al., 2019).

13.4.5 Data Analysis Techniques

A broad range of data is collected from the integrated source of IoMT and ML devices. Several techniques of data analysis are applied to derive these insights. The approaches range over various approaches, such as anomaly detection, clustering, classification, and predictive modeling. Predictive modeling predicts further outcomes based on past data, thereby allowing proactive healthcare interventions. There are specific techniques for finding anomalies in patterns which are a must for catching abnormalities or possible health hazards early. Apart from this, various algorithms are used for clustering, bringing similar data points together to assist with treatment plans tailored to every patient. In addition, classification algorithms help split data into disjoint groups to make work easier in tasks like drug prescription or disease diagnosis. Combining these strategies enable integration of IoMT and ML devices to enhance patient outcomes, optimize resource use, and deliver improvements in healthcare services (Giri et al., 2019).

13.4.6 Ethical Considerations

In most cases, ethical considerations take the upper-hand, and hence during the development and deployment of new techniques in the healthcare industry, especially during the involvement of IoMT and ML devices. In order to ensure ethical considerations, there is a need for implementation of access controls, anonymization methods, and strong encryption protocols that can protect data privacy and security which could ensure confidentiality and availability. With this, fairness along with the reduction of biases is important and can be achieved through factors like algorithmic decision-making, transparency, and accountability. Mechanisms must also be put into place regarding consent, so individuals can give informed consent for the collection, storage, and use of their health information. In addition to the above, the IoMT systems should be continually monitored and reviewed to enhance their efficiency and to answer ethical requirements (Char et al., 2020).

13.4.7 Limitations of Methodology

Although ML and IoMT technologies have the potential to completely transform healthcare, there are still several barriers that must be removed in order to improve performance and accuracy, which will enable IoMT establish a foothold in the sector. The primary drawback is that issues including sensor accuracy, signal noise, and incompleteness can impair the quality and dependability of data gathered from IoMT devices. The second issue is the interpretability of machine learning models, which can be problematic in some situations and make algorithmic recommendations hard for medical professionals to understand. Concerns about data security and privacy are another major issue since sharing private health data among IoMT devices increases the possibility of misuse, data breaches, and illegal access. Disparate data formats, standards, and compatibility issues hinder scalability and interoperability in IoMT and ML. Concerns about algorithmic bias, autonomy, and consent necessitate ongoing ethical analysis and regulation. Interdisciplinary cooperation, technology advancement, and policy intervention can work together to lessen the difficulties (Kamalov et al., 2023).

13.4.8 Conclusion and Summary

To put it briefly, the combination of IoMT and ML approaches gives a revolutionary expectation in the healthcare sector, offering a customized viewpoint in addition to improved and precise patient outcomes. This clever tactic nevertheless has shortcomings that must be addressed. This includes problems with data quality, interpretability, privacy, scalability, and moral dilemmas, to name but a few. These challenges underscore the necessity of careful consideration and ongoing development (Hireche et al., 2022). In order to make IoMT and ML a part of success stories in the healthcare industry, this study attempts to investigate the elements that prevent technology from improving and, conversely, the factors that could be improved.

13.5 FINDINGS AND RESULTS

13.5.1 Introduction to Findings and Results

This study presents the key findings involved in the success stories and advancements in healthcare through IoMT and ML. The results and findings are organized as per the objectives mentioned in the introduction. Findings provided in this section are the key reasons for either success or failure of IoMT and ML devices based on the factors like performance, quality, security, ethical considerations, and other factors.

13.5.2 Key Factors for Success Stories of IoMT and ML

The IoMT collaboration with ML brought a revolution in healthcare industry. The IoMT made it possible by its capability to collect the real-time data from patients, medical devices, and facilities. This IoMT which greatly empowered early intervention and individualized treatment plans is made possible by the data's ability to monitor vital signs, medication compliance, and disease progression remotely. This proved that utilization of IoMT devices can lead to proactive care, better patient outcomes, and fewer readmissions to hospitals by giving healthcare providers access to timely insights. This feature of IoMT is considered as the first advantageous step to the success stories ("copperdigital", 2024).

Second, IoMT devices' interconnectedness and interoperability improve stakeholder communication and care coordination. IoMT devices facilitate the sharing of patient data and medical information across multiple healthcare settings, thereby promoting continuity of care and minimizing administrative burdens. This is made possible by their seamless integration with EHRs and other clinical systems. Healthcare professionals are better able to work together as multidisciplinary care teams and make decisions that are well-informed and grounded in comprehensive patient data because of this interoperability ("copperdigital", 2024).

Additionally, IoMT devices promote patient's empowerment and engagement by enabling self-management and remote monitoring capabilities. Patients are able to take an active role in their care by monitoring their health metrics, accessing educational materials, and interacting with their healthcare providers through wearable technology and mobile apps. Patients are better able to take charge of their health and follow their treatment plans when proactive healthcare is provided, which in return improves patient satisfaction and health outcomes ("copperdigital", 2024).

IoMT devices also aid in cost reduction and improved operational effectiveness for healthcare institutions. IoMT devices contribute to lower administrative overhead and higher productivity by automating repetitive tasks, optimizing resource utilization, and streamlining workflows. Furthermore, IoMT-enabled machine learning and predictive analytics algorithms find ways to optimize processes, allocate resources more efficiently, and save costs—all of which help healthcare providers provide high-quality care at a reasonable cost. These are key findings of IoMT involved in the success stories in the domain of healthcare ("copperdigital", 2024).

13.5.3 Key Features for IoMT Preference over Other Technologies

The combination of IoMT and ML is preferred over alternative technologies for a number of important reasons that work together to improve healthcare delivery. First, it is the ability of IoMT to generate a massive volume of data from a multitude of sources, including wearable technology, medical sensors, and EHRs. ML algorithms are excellent at finding patterns, trends, and insights that can guide clinical decision-making when it comes to examining vast and intricate datasets. IoMT devices can predict patient outcomes, make more accurate diagnoses, and customize treatment plans based on unique patient characteristics and medical histories by utilizing ML to extract actionable intelligence from raw data ("ET Special", 2023).

Second, ML-supported IoMT devices have predictive capacities which in turn help making proactive and preventive healthcare interventions possible. ML algorithms can detect early warning indicators of worsening health conditions by analyzing real-time sensor readings and historical patient data. This ability allows for prompt interventions to avert unfavorable events and hospitalizations. The predictive modeling capability enhances patient outcomes and lowers healthcare costs related to avoidable complications by enabling healthcare providers to transition from reactive to proactive care delivery ("ET Special", 2023).

Additionally, IoMT devices promote patient empowerment and engagement by enabling self-management and remote monitoring capabilities. Patients can take an active role in their care by monitoring their health metrics, accessing educational materials, and interacting with their healthcare providers through wearable technology and mobile apps. Patients are better able to take charge of their health and follow their treatment plans when proactive healthcare is provided, which improves patient satisfaction and health outcomes ("ET Special", 2023).

The integration of IoMT with ML has the potential to provide personalized medicine approaches as the ML algorithms has the ability to analyze multi-modal data streams, including genetic, environmental, and lifestyle factors. Along with this, the ML algorithms have the capability to identify patient-specific risk factors, treatment responses, and disease trajectories. As a result, it puts healthcare providers at ease as they can deliver targeted interventions and therapies, maximizing treatment efficacy and minimizing adverse effects. This is also a major feature which contributes to the success stories in the healthcare industry. These are some other factors responsible for preferring IoMT over other technologies ("ET Special", 2023).

13.5.4 Limitations of IoMT: A Cause of Failure of Success Stories

The shortcomings of IoMT have in fact played a role in some of the failure stories. The interoperability problem is one major drawback. IoMT devices frequently use different communication protocols which are made by different manufacturers causing compatibility problems and making it difficult to integrate them into the healthcare systems that are already in place. The inability of devices and healthcare platforms to exchange data can cause disruptions in care coordination and undermine the efficacy of IoMT solutions. IoMT initiatives may face obstacles to their success. Healthcare professionals would not be able to obtain critical information required for making informed clinical decisions, for example, if the data from a wearable fitness tracker could not be smoothly synchronized with a patient's EHR system (Petersen-Khmelnitski, 2024).

Another limitation is the concern for data security and privacy. Patients' vital signs, medical histories, and personal identification numbers are collected via IoMT devices. Therefore, if these data are not well protected, they may be vulnerable to abuse, unauthorized access, and data breaches, which could jeopardize patient confidentiality and confidence. The realization of the potential benefits of IoMT solutions can be hampered by instances of data breaches or privacy violations which can undermine patient confidence in these solutions and discourage healthcare organizations from investing in or implementing them (Kamalov et al., 2023).

Moreover, the precision and reliability of an IoMT device can be its greatest disadvantage. Many IoMT devices rely on wireless communication and sensors to collect and transmit data. The accuracy and reliability of the data collected may be compromised if these sensors are not calibrated correctly or if there are connectivity issues. This could lead to inaccurate clinical interpretations and subpar patient care. For example, diabetic individuals may receive the incorrect dosage of insulin and suffer adverse health effects if a wearable glucose monitor provides misleading results (Garg et al., 2022). Moreover, regulatory obstacles and compliance needs can also make IoMT projects less successful. The IoMT's efficacy, safety, and adherence to healthcare laws are required to be guaranteed, hence strict regulatory standards and approval procedures apply to medical devices, including IoMT devices. For device makers and healthcare providers, navigating these regulatory obstacles can be time- and resource-consuming which delays the implementation of IoMT solutions and prevents their widespread adoption. The mitigation of these challenges can prevent failure of IoMT models (Petersen-Khmelnitski, 2024).

13.5.5 Conclusion and Summary

In summary, the success of IoMT is guaranteed by key features like personalized healthcare delivery, interoperability, real-time data collection, and remote monitoring capabilities. IoMT can be hindered in its effectiveness and adoption by a number of limitations, including complexities related to regulations, data security, interoperability, and reliability. Stakeholders need to put a high priority on standardization to enhance device accuracy and reliability, strengthen cybersecurity, and expedite regulatory procedures in order to lessen these constraints. IoMT can reach its full potential in revolutionizing patient outcomes and healthcare delivery by resolving these issues.

13.6 DISCUSSION

13.6.1 Introduction to Discussion

This study focused on the key factors responsible for success of IoMT model in collaboration with ML algorithms. The discussion sections will unveil some real-time incidents as case studies to provide more insight into success and advancement of IoMT in integration with ML. This discussion will cover all the mentioned criteria in introduction and stand out as supportive theory for research findings.

13.6.2 Case Study 1: Predictive Maintenance in Medical Imaging Equipment

In the medical imaging field, building new technologies that have sensors embedded in CT and MRI scanners enables automatic detection, diagnosis, and treatment of a wide variety of diseases in a timely manner. Unfortunately, placing new medical imaging equipment is expensive, and the unexpected breakdowns can impede patient care, bear high repair charges, and even deter productivity, leading to undesirable monetary implications. In light of this, the researchers attached IoMT devices equipped with sensors to medical imaging devices to address this issue by continuously tracking and assessing performance and operational parameters in real time. Moreover, these sensors combine to allow for monitoring of vibration, temperature, power consumption, as well as usage trends, ensuring seamless data flow and feedback. Most importantly, having an abundance of data serves as an edge for this technology as mounting insightful information accelerates strategizing to mitigate problems and irregularities. The amalgamation of sensor and historical data assists in training machine learning algorithms to not only detect patterns but also evaluate relations suggesting likely breakdowns of equipment. By identifying patterns with trends in historical data, these ML models can predict when the components of medical devices may deteriorate or fail. This ultimately assists in deploying preemptive maintenance actions before greater problems ensue. So, to avoid any proactive maintenance interventions moving forward, this allows for planning to take place. This problem is also mitigated by the integration of IoMT and ML which facilitates decision-making and resource allocation in healthcare settings. Insights gained through predictive maintenance can help the healthcare experts to manage the medically important resources well by extending the life of expensive equipment, setting their prioritization, and planning for maintenance routines. This ensures that critical diagnostic tools and other resources are efficient and dependable, which then positively impacts on the care and treatment of the patients. Overall, this case study demonstrates that IoMT and ML can revolutionize the historical methods of maintaining the medical imaging equipment. They help medical providers reduce costs, enhance the quality and continuity of care, and make maintenance of the equipment more proactive by utilizing predictive analytics (Perea G.H, 2020).

13.6.3 Case Study 2:

Remote Patient Monitoring Using Wearable Sensors and Machine Learning—A Case Study in Parkinson's disease

This particular case report is based on the application of ML algorithms together with wearable sensors in supervising Parkinson's disease patients remotely. Parkinson's disease is a progressive disorder of the CNS that affects movement and includes bradykinesia, rigidity, and tremors among other movement symptoms. To ensure treatment is effective and results are improved, it is necessary to keep an eye on the symptoms and on how they develop over time. These sensors provided unbiased data streams about the frequency and intensity of patients' motor symptoms in real time. Patients were also asked to perform some standardized motor exercises such as a finger-tap and a gait test in order to obtain particular motor markers for Parkinson's disease. Once the data from the sensors was collected, the data was processed and analyzed using algorithms that were trained with machine learning to be able to detect patterns indicating the presence of Parkinson's disease symptoms. The algorithms also extracted various features from the sensor data and were able to integrate various signal processing techniques to categorize the motor data into bradykinesia, dyskinesia, and resting tremor motor states. A series of machine learning algorithms were trained to accurately identify and quantify the motor signs of patients with Parkinson's disease using the features obtained from the sensors and the clinical evaluations done by specialists in movement disorders. Moreover, this research indicated that the use of wearable sensors and the implementation of ML algorithms could enable effective remote monitoring of patients with Parkinson's disease. For instance, patients would benefit from proper management of motor symptoms without having to frequently visit clinical settings for evaluation.

13.6.4 Case Study 3:

Smart Hospital Infrastructure Optimization

In demonstrating the areas where the efficiency of the hospital can be enhanced, machine learning algorithms and the IoMT devices are good examples to consider. The primary objective of this research is to improve the overall quality of care given to the patient by way of optimizing the infrastructure and resources of the hospital so that the expenses are kept at the minimum and efficiency is at the max. The research then places sensors throughout the hospital, in particular inside patient rooms, operating rooms, ER, and diagnostic . Furthermore, the devices embedded in the sensors allow gathering data in real time regarding patient traffic, occupancy, equipment usage, and environmental settings. For instance, these devices are equipped with a number of sensors which enable tracking movement of the patients and the staff together with measuring temperature, humidity, and air quality levels. The implementation of ML algorithms of varying complexity in the phase, including data gathering from IoMT devices, helps defining patterns, trends, and correlations in the data collected. For instance, the use of predictive models based on machine learning enables managers to analyze the flow of patients and determine the busiest times of the week for each service. The research indicates the potential for ML interpretations to be turned into actionable strategies that can improve the functioning of the hospital and its services. For instance, the hospital managers may alter the staffing rosters or the layout of the patient wards in an effort to reduce wait time and maximize patient throughput, as recommended through ML insights concerning patient flow patterns. Along similar lines, ML techniques can also help in identifying the equipment or facilities which are currently underutilized and would benefit from capital improvements or the installation of new equipment, thereby enhancing capacity and meeting the increasing market demand. All the aspects of the case study support the ability to incorporate IoMTs with ML technologies in healthcare settings. It is proved that the inclusion of real data, algorithms, and the optimization of infrastructure and resources assist hospitals to build up the effectiveness and the quality of the process of patient care services. This approach not only enhances the overall quality of healthcare for the patients (Z. Chaczko; et al., 2010), but also helps healthcare institutions reduce their operational costs and improve efficiency during frequent changes across the healthcare environment.

13.6.5 Case Study 4:

Early Detection of Sepsis in Intensive Care Units—A Machine Learning Case Study

As illustrated in the case study, ML algorithms are utilized to detect signs of early sepsis in individuals who have been admitted to the intensive care units (ICUs). It is important to note that sepsis is a condition that occurs as a result of an infection and a disorganized immune response that can be endorsed to a life-threatening complication. In this particular case, a sepsis diagnosis can be facilitated using ML algorithms that are trained on patient data obtained via vital signs alongside lab tests, clinical notes, and patient records. Each patient's time spent in an ICU facilitates the identification of sepsis and correlating stressors. Once relevant patterns are established, ML models can then utilize real-time patient data collected from monitoring devices in conjunction with EHRs in critical care settings. This pre-emptive method of training the ML models aids in distinguishing minor changes in patient clinical markers that could indicate the presence of sepsis. More importantly, the ML algorithm has the ability to continuously monitor patient data and spot trends that are more likely to endorse sepsis prior to clinical symptoms being apparent. The research depicts how early diagnosis and treatment of sepsis, if ML becomes a part of the solution, can be lifesaving and substantially lower the sepsis-related morbidity and mortality rates. For example, the ML algorithms can track a patient who is about to develop sepsis and inform the medical team that antibiotics or fluids are needed together with intensive surveillance of the patient for any signs of deterioration. The research also points out that it is continuously learning that AL and ML systems have such an outstanding ability to refresh themselves and their functions as well, and this is more than the ability to memorize things. For instance, machine learning models' prediction accuracy improves as they are exposed to an evolving array of patients. This change provides greater reliability to the model's ability to detect early onset of sepsis infection. Continuous learning also contributes to the optimization of patient management by ensuring that health professionals remain aware of shifts in trends. In summary, there is evidence from the case study that ML models for earlier sepsis detection in an ICU environment can bring benefits with respect to both ease of use and time saving. Providers will be able to better manage real-time patient information, lower costs, and provide more efficient service in ICUs.

13.6.6 Case Study 5:

Personalized Treatment Recommendations in Oncology—Integrating Machine Learning with Clinical Decision Support Systems

This chapter aims to evaluate the integration of clinical decision support systems alongside ML. It focuses on how these systems and algorithms can match patients suffering from cancer with cancer treatment stimulation systems. It further mentions the use of data including demographics of the patients, histology of the tumors, genetic information, and other contributing clinical details. This data is then employed in training algorithms based on ML. EHRs, medical imaging, genomic data, and treatment registers are also utilized to select the required data when designing models that focus on the prediction of treatment outcomes. Furthermore, it assists in decision-making regarding the models for treatment when they have undergone training. Clinical decision support systems integrate the models and assist oncologists in providing the recommendation to the patients while evaluating their clinical and tumor information. The ML algorithms developed earlier are then used to provide the patients suffering from cancer with a critical diagnosis. Some types of target therapy and chemo are often included in the recommendation provided. Zdorovie's study demonstrates oncologist Zvonarev's use of deep neural networks that suggest personalized treatment recommendations to each cancer patient. This study is of crucial importance as personalized care is a novel approach that promises big advantages with respect to patient satisfaction and therapy outcomes, aimed at individualizing the approach to the very selecting of the therapy type and to the very precise targeting of the treatment. The chapter recalls and explains why cancer evolution is no longer enough to just analyze and adjust occurrence of a particular mutation or position in the genome to devise an effective treatment using ML algorithms. These capabilities allow system users to learn from and address feedback, allowing the user to rapidly adopt new technologies, methodologies, and treatments. The simultaneous integration of advanced medical technology, computer science tools, and deep level understanding of patient evolution in their healthcare needs provides the incentive to rethink and establish effective cancer treatment plans that both ensure efficiency and great therapy outcomes. Innovations in deep neural networks are revolutionizing the way analytics can be used to make more effective and precise the construction of therapeutic strategies aimed at combating the disease. The study shows step by step how the deep neural networks used by Zvonarev and his team can reconstruct therapeutic approaches and predict treatment options for new patients.

13.6.7 Conclusion and Summary

To wrap it up, the results assimilated after reviewing a few case studies demonstrated the contribution of IoMT into the healthcare industry, indicating that IoMT played a pivotal role in revolutionizing the healthcare ecosystem. Also, it is shown by this particular research that IoMT has already been embedded into the medical field from low-tier devices to high-end applications. However, in order for IoMT to survive in the healthcare industry, it is crucial to address some of the existing challenges as well as forecast the potential challenges that lie ahead.

13.7 CONCLUSION

13.7.1 Restating Findings

In conclusion, this study has unveiled the key factors responsible for the success of IoMT and ML architecture. In addition, the limitations which caused failure of models or that could cause failure are put forward with supportive explanations. The factors that stand out as hindrance are notified and importance for mitigation of the issues is provided along with impacts and destructions that cause if not mitigated.

13.7.2 Revisiting the Objectives

The study addressed the research objectives of unveiling the success stories and advancements in healthcare through IoMT with real incidents and case studies as the center of attraction, identifying the wealth of IoMT over other existing technology, unleash the key reasons and backstories of IoMT's success stories and advancements, and proposing future research direction and recommendations for maximizing the benefits of IoMT in integration with ML.

13.7.3 Implications of Findings

The findings of this study have vital inference for theory, practice, and policy in domain of healthcare. From theoretical perspective, the results produced contributes to the better understanding of IoMT role in advancement in healthcare and how the IoMT as technology evolved itself with the support of ML algorithms. By discussing various case studies, the key reasons behind the success stories along with limitation to be addressed are well-described theoretically.

13.7.4 Practical Recommendations

Based on the findings, several recommendations for practical implementation are mentioned. In addition, the advancements and growth that could be achieved by mitigating security-related issues and interoperability issues are also discussed. The more training of ML algorithms can produce more accurate results allowing health providers with easy diagnosis process without any delay.

13.7.5 Theoretical Contributions

This study contributes to theoretical understanding by providing factual evidence supporting the influence of IoMT and contribution of IoMT to advancement and improved performance of healthcare industry. The findings discussed in the study provide a basement for future research on IoMT with ML in healthcare. Furthermore, the study highlights the significance of ethical considerations, security, privacy, and accuracy for a successful IoMT implementation in healthcare.

13.7.6 Limitations and Future Directions

Despite the advantages, there are certain limitations that need be noted. The retrospective process of data collection may lead to missing data and documentation errors which could compromise the findings generalizability. Further studies should use multi-center trials and longitudinal studies to conclusively identify the effectiveness of IoMT technologies in a range of healthcare environments. This will ensure responsible IoMT deployment in integration with ML in healthcare integrating research on sociable and ethical issues related to IoMT, such as accountability, equity, and transparency.

13.7.7 Final Thoughts and Closing Remarks

To summarize the study, IoMT devices and ML applications have a wide set of areas in the healthcare world. Clinical IoT can revolutionize the way medical care is provided to people by enhancing theory-driven diagnosis and improving clinical processes. However, to fully benefit from IoMT and ML integration in clinical practice, concerns about algorithm bias, data consent, and safety should be resolved. Further studies and partnerships are essential in order to take full advantage of IoMT and ML technologies to improve healthcare systems and outcomes globally.

13.8 FUTURE DIRECTIONS FOR RESEARCH

13.8.1 Introduction to Future Directions

The findings and discussion of this study provide significant insights into the influence of IoMT to ameliorate diagnostic accuracy and patient outcomes in healthcare. Further, there is a need for future investigation to advance knowledge, stay updated, and address the remaining gaps in the field of IoMT in the healthcare industry.

13.8.2 Identification of Research Gaps

One area for future research is to explore the long-term impact of IoMT devices and ML-assisted diagnostic algorithms on patient outcomes, including clinical outcomes, patient satisfactory, healthcare utilization, and outcome accuracy. This study demonstrated need for improvements in diagnostic accuracy security along with the key factors of successful model. Still, there is a need for further research to assess implications of IoMT and ML integration on patient care processes and healthcare delivery.

13.8.3 Integration with Existing Literature

Future research should expand the existing literature on IoMT collaboration with ML in healthcare, extending current knowledge and addressing remaining research gaps leading to identification of theoretical and practical framework that could create a basement for success stories of IoMT in healthcare industry.

13.8.4 Methodological Considerations

Methodological considerations for future research include the development of strong designs for study, data collection methods, analytical approaches along with longitudinal and multi-centered trials which are required to evaluate the long-term impact of IoMT and ML integration in healthcare, while the qualitative research methods can provide insights into user experiences and socio-technical dynamics of IoMT implementation.

13.8.5 Potential Research Questions

Proposed research questions for future investigation:

1. How does IoMT's integration with ML impact clinical decision-making processes and patient outcome in healthcare industry?
2. What are the factors that stand as barriers or hindrance in the failed real-time IoMT model?
3. How IoMT technologies can be effectively integrated into existing cybersecurity tools to protect privacy, confidentiality, integrity, and availability of medical data?
4. What are the possible mitigations to protect the ethical and societal consideration of IoMT?

13.8.6 Ethical and Societal Considerations

Ethical and societal considerations such as patient privacy, data security, algorithmic bias, and informed consent are factors that greatly influence the development and deployment of IoMT technologies in healthcare. Future research should give importance to addressing the mitigation for security issues for medical data.

13.8.7 Conclusion and Summary

In conclusion, future research in IoMT-driven healthcare holds promising role in improving diagnostic accuracy, patient outcomes, and healthcare delivery. Researchers can advance knowledge and contribute to the evolution of IoMT to create a revolution in healthcare industry by addressing identified gaps, collaborating interdisciplinary perspectives, and leveraging emerging technologies.

REFERENCES

Bgosoftware. (2024, February 2). 10 Internet of Things (IoT) Healthcare Examples. Retrieved from https://www.bgosoftware.com/blog/10-internet-of-things-iot-healthcare-examples/#:~:text=Wearable%20devices%20such%20as%20smartwatches%2C%20phones%2C%20or%20wearable%20sensors%20automatically,body%2Dfat%20percentage%2C%20etc

Brena, R. F., Aguileta, A. A., Trejo, L. A., Molino-Minero-Re, E., & Mayora, O. (2020). Choosing the Best Sensor Fusion Method: A Machine-Learning Approach. *Sensors (Basel)*, 20(8), 2350. https://doi.org/10.3390/s20082350

Char, D. S., Abràmoff, M. D., & Feudtner, C. (2020). Identifying Ethical Considerations for Machine Learning Healthcare Applications. *The American Journal of Bioethics*, 20(11), 7–17. https://doi.org/10.1080/15265161.2020.1819469

Copperdigital. (2024). The Impact of the Internet of Medical Things on the Healthcare Industry. Retrieved February 18, 2024, from https://copperdigital.com/blog/internet-of-medical-things-overview/

Dwivedi, R., Mehrotra, D., & Chandra, S. (2022). Potential of Internet of Medical Things (IoMT) Applications in Building a Smart Healthcare System: A Systematic Review. *Journal of Oral Biology and Craniofacial Research*, 12(2), 302–318. https://doi.org/10.1016/j.jobcr.2021.11.010

ET Special. (2023, August 18). Enhancing Medical Services: How Internet and IoMT are Shaping Healthcare. *The Economic Times*. Retrieved from https://m.economictimes.com/jobs/mid-career/enhancing-medical-services-how-internet-and-iomt-are-shaping-healthcare/articleshow/102836560.cms

Firican, G. (2024). The History of Machine Learning. *Lights on Data*. Retrieved February 8, 2024, from https://www.lightsondata.com/the-history-of-machine-learning/

Garg, N., Wazid, M., Singh, J., Singh, D. P., & Das, A. K. (2022, May 15). Security in IoMT-driven Smart Healthcare: A Comprehensive Review and Open Challenges. *Healthcare Security and Privacy*. https://doi.org/10.1002/spy2.235

Giri, A., Chatterjee, S., Paul, P., Chakraborty, S., & Biswas, S. (2019). Impact of 'Smart Applications of IoMT (Internet of Medical Things)' on Health-Care Domain in India. *International Journal of Recent Technology and Engineering (IJRTE)*, 8, 881–885. HTTPS://DOI.ORG/10.35940/ijrte.D7474.118419.

Hireche, R., Mansouri, H., & Pathan, A.-S. K. (2022). Security and Privacy Management in Internet of Medical Things (IoMT): A Synthesis. *Journal of Cybersecurity and Privacy*, 2(3), 640–661. https://doi.org/10.3390/jcp2030033

IoT.Business.News. (2023, June 12). Transforming Healthcare through IoMT Firmware Development. *IoT Business News*. https://iotbusinessnews.com/2023/06/12/64365-transforming-healthcare-through-iomt-firmware-development/

Kamalov, F., Pourghebleh, B., Gheisari, M., Liu, Y., & Moussa, S. (2023). Internet of Medical Things Privacy and Security: Challenges, Solutions, and Future Trends from a New Perspective. *Sustainability*, 15(4), 3317. https://doi.org/10.3390/su15043317

Lutkevich, B., & DelVecchio, A. (2024). Internet of Medical Things (IoMT) or Healthcare IoT. *TechTarget*. Retrieved February 8, 2024, from https://www.techtarget.com/iotagenda/definition/IoMT-Internet-of-Medical-Things

Merchant, N. (2024). What is the Internet of Things? Vision of Humanity. *World Economic Forum*. Retrieved February 8, 2024, from https://www.visionofhumanity.org/what-is-the-internet-of-things/

Miliard, M. (2023, August 30). Safeguarding IoMT and Connected Devices is an Ongoing Challenge. *Healthcare IT News*. Retrieved from https://www.healthcareitnews.com/news/safeguarding-iomt-and-connected-devices-ongoing-challenge

Nigar, N., Jaleel, A., Islam, S., Shahzad, M. K., & Affum, E. A. (2023). IoMT Meets Machine Learning: From Edge to Cloud Chronic Diseases Diagnosis System. *Journal of Healthcare Engineering*, 2023(Article ID 9995292), 13 pages. https://doi.org/10.1155/2023/9995292

Ordr. (2024). 10 Internet of Things (IoT) Healthcare Examples, and Why Their Security Matters. Retrieved February 12, 2024, from https://ordr.net/article/iot-healthcare-examples/

Perea, G. H., (2020). *Predictive Maintenance in Medical Imaging Equipment: A Case Study. Journal of Medical Systems*. 44(2), 1-13

Petersen-Khmelnitski, L. (2024). Internet of Medical Things: Challenges and Adoptions. *CIFS Health*. Retrieved February 18, 2024, from https://cifs.health/backgrounds/internet-of-medical-things-challenges-and-adoptions

Prasad, V. K., Bhattacharya, P., Maru, D., Tanwar, S., Verma, A., Singh, A., Tiwari, A. K., Sharma, R., Alkhayyat, A., Ţurcanu, F.-E., et al. (2023). Federated Learning for the Internet-of-Medical-Things: A Survey. *Mathematics*, 11(1), 151. https://doi.org/10.3390/math11010151

Razdan, S., & Sharma, S. (2022). Internet of Medical Things (IoMT): Overview, Emerging Technologies, and Case Studies. *IETE Technical Review*, 39(4), 775–788. HTTPS://DOI.ORG/10.1080/02564602.2021.1927863

Sadhu, P. K., Yanambaka, V. P., Abdelgawad, A., & Yelamarthi, K. (2022). Prospect of Internet of Medical Things: A Review on Security Requirements and Solutions. *Sensors (Basel)*, 22(15), 5517. https://doi.org/10.3390/s22155517

Shafiq, M., Choi, J.-G., Cheikhrouhou, O., & Hamam, H. (2024). Advances in IoMT for Healthcare Systems. *Sensors*, 24(1), 10. https://doi.org/10.3390/s24010010

Shakeel, T., Habib, S., Boulila, W., Koubaa, A., Javed, A. R., Rizwan, M., Gadekallu, T. R., & Sufiyan, M. (2023). A Survey on COVID-19 Impact in the Healthcare Domain: Worldwide Market Implementation, Applications, Security and Privacy Issues, Challenges and Future Prospects. *Complex Intelligent Systems*, 9(1), 1027–1058. HTTPS://DOI.ORG/10.1007/s40747-022-00767-w. Erratum in: Complex Intelligent Systems, 2022 Oct 17:1. PMID: 35668731; PMCID: PMC9151356.

Srivastava, J., Routray, S., Ahmad, S., & Waris, M. M. (2022). Internet of Medical Things (IoMT)-Based Smart Healthcare System: Trends and Progress. *Computational Intelligence and Neuroscience*, 2022, 7218113. https://doi.org/10.1155/2022/7218113. Retraction in: Computational Intelligence and Neuroscience, 2023, 9768292. PMID: 35880061; PMCID: PMC9308524.

Suresh Babu, C. V., Akkash Anniyappa, C. S., Karthik, A. S., Babu, S., Pavan, Y. S., & Brahanandam, C. B. (2024). Equity-Driven Solutions: Harnessing IoT Technology to Mitigate Health Risks and Bridge Gaps in E-Waste Management. In R. K. V., H. Kannan, D. Spodarets, P. Khan, & B. Pradhan (Eds.), *Sustainable Solutions for E-Waste and Development* (pp. 146–163). IGI Global. https://doi.org/10.4018/979-8-3693-1018-2.ch011

Suresh Babu, C. V., Akshayah, N. S., & Maclin Vinola, P. (2024). Artificial Intelligence in Healthcare: Assessing Impacts, Challenges, and Recommendations for Achieving Healthcare Independence. In N. Geada & G. Jamil (Eds.), *Perspectives on Artificial Intelligence in Times of Turbulence: Theoretical Background to Applications* (pp. 61–80). IGI Global. https://doi.org/10.4018/978-1-6684-9814-9.ch005

Suresh Babu, C. V., & Praveen, S. (2023). Swarm Intelligence and Evolutionary Machine Learning Algorithms for COVID-19: Pandemic and Epidemic Review. In A. Suresh Kumar, U. Kose, S. Sharma, & S. Jerald Nirmal Kumar (Eds.), *Dynamics of Swarm Intelligence Health Analysis for the Next Generation* (pp. 83–103). IGI Global. https://doi.org/10.4018/978-1-6684-6894-4.ch005

Thaploo, V. (2023, July 9). Internet of Medical Things (IoMT) in e-clinics: Enabling connected healthcare in smart cities. *Voices, Lifestyle, TOI.* Retrieved from https://timesofindia.indiatimes.com/blogs/voices/internet-of-medical-things-iomt-in-e-clinics-enabling-connected-healthcare-in-smart-cities/

Vishnu, S., Ramson, S. R. J., & Jegan, R. (2020). Internet of Medical Things (IoMT) - An overview. In *2020 5th International Conference on Devices, Circuits and Systems (ICDCS)* (pp. 101–104). Coimbatore, India. https://doi.org/10.1109/ICDCS48716.2020.243558

Watts, S. (2023, November 13). The Internet of Medical Things (IoMT): A Brief Introduction. Retrieved from https://www.splunk.com/en_us/blog/learn/the-internet-of-medical-things-iomt.html

Z. Chaczko; C. Chiu; A.S. Kohli; V. Mahadevan; (2010) *Smart Hospital Management System: an integration of enterprise level solutions utilising open group architecture framework, International Conference on Computer Science and Information Technology,* Vol.5, pp. 8-15

Index

For Product Safety Concerns and Information please contact our EU representative GPSR@taylorandfrancis.com
Taylor & Francis Verlag GmbH, Kaufingerstraße 24, 80331 München, Germany

www.ingramcontent.com/pod-product-compliance
Ingram Content Group UK Ltd.
Pitfield, Milton Keynes, MK11 3LW, UK
UKHW020201200926
475702UK00004B/562
* 9 7 8 1 0 3 2 7 4 8 9 3 1 *